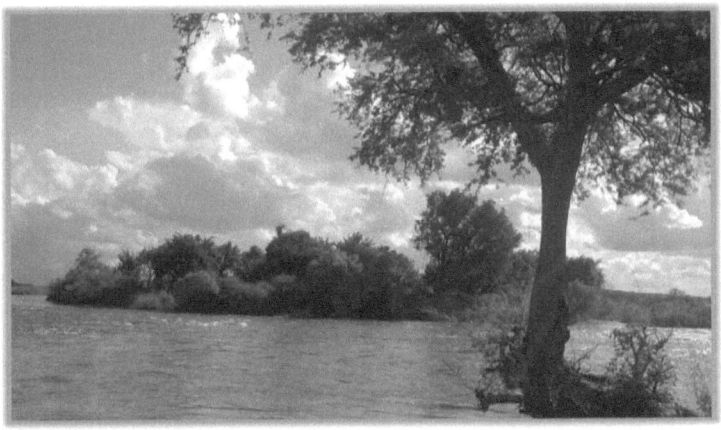

"A physician is not angry at the intemperance of a mad patient, nor does he take it ill to be railed at by a man in fever. Just so should a wise man treat all mankind, as a physician does his patient, and look upon them only as sick and extravagant."

Lucius

Annaeus Seneca

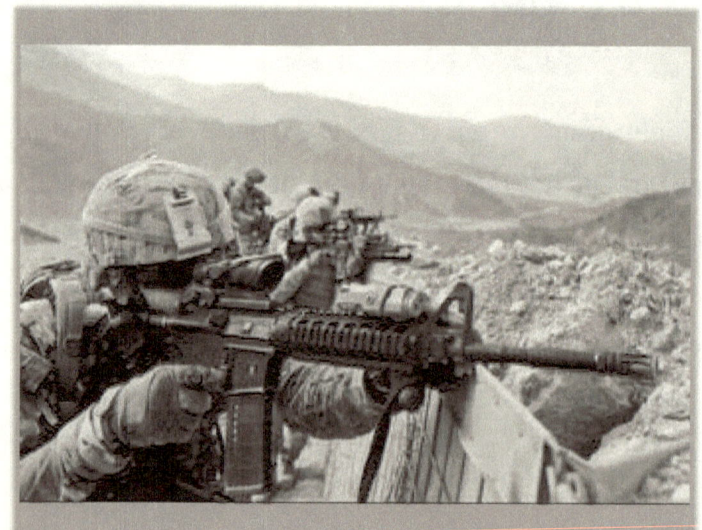

"Given one well-trained physician of the highest type he will do better work for a thousand people than ten specialists."

William J. Mayo

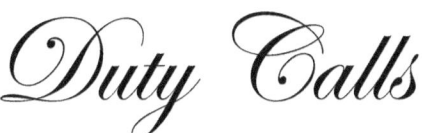

Duty Calls

People pay the doctor for his trouble; for his kindness they still remain in his debt.

Seneca

Inspired by a True Life Story

Dr Kelvin C Moonga

DEDICATION

This book is dedicated to my patients, past present and future.

To

Jay, John, Joshua and Matildah

Whose laughter I missed dearly during the writing of this book

&

Victoria

My mother Pauline

For introducing me to the art of storytelling and for teaching me
how to read many years ago

My Father, J M Moonga

For his wise counsel that set me on a Career in Medicine

And

My readers for encouraging me to write this book

INTRODUCTION

Choosing a well paying Career can be a daunting task for someone slothful. Long hours of dedication to study and to master the necessary skills will invariably demand personal sacrifice. Unfortunately it appears Studies alone and acquisition of Degrees is not an answer to success.

The race is not to the swift or the battle to the strong, nor does food come to the wise or wealth to the brilliant or favor to the learned; but time and chance happen to them all. Or put simply, the fastest runner doesn't always win the race, and the strongest warrior doesn't always win the battle. The wise sometimes go hungry, and the skillful are not necessarily wealthy. And those who are educated don't always lead successful lives. It is all decided by chance, by being in the right place at the right time. Ecclesiastes 9:11.

Often many accept to undertake certain Duties for monetary gain. In the world today, the more Herculean the task, the less the pay... The man toiling on the land to feed his nation receives less pay compared to the middle man engaged in trading off the produce of the laborer's sweat. The middle man took his chances to avoid the land and chose his timing.

When Duty Calls to report an emergency such as a Life and death matter; or simply a case of someone caught between a rock and a hard place; a passerby maybe all that Time and Chance brings to the fore.

There are often no terms and conditions attached to answering Life's Duty Calls; from as little as picking a Child's favourite Toy and returning it to the kid who lost it to lending a hand at a horrific accident scene; monetary gain is often not part of the motivating factors in accepting the Call. **What is at stake is often priceless**;

Table of Contents

Difficult Decisions

My skirmish with state house begun on a not so ordinary Lusaka Friday afternoon while conducting a routine ward round at 5pm. I met Mulenga in the special Maternity unit were she had been admitted for four days. I learnt from her file that she was being treated for malaria and intra uterine fetal death.

I was the only one who didn't know that her father was a minister at State House.

The turnover of ministers had been too high that I could hardly keep up to date with their names, let alone their children. This particular minister was the president's first cousin. That meant she was the president's niece. Her uncle was a very terrifying statesman, especially when you happen to be on the wrong side of the law. He would ensure the long arm of the law visited you.

That morning I arrived late at the hospital and missed the hand over round.

My landlord was moving back into her house, which meant I was homeless. I had 24hrs to find alternative accommodation and a busy

Friday call waiting for me.

Life in Lusaka had become very expensive, rentals were sky rocketing. Call day was the busiest shift at the Hospital. I chose to work, even when I could have decided to stay away, in order to prepare my mind on an impending odious house hunt and shifting awaiting me

When I finally caught up with the team, I quickly presented my 'shelter predicaments' to them. But no one showed any profound empathy. I knew some of them had been through this before and so it wasn't news.

Mulenga had been referred to the University Hospital at the end of October from a private clinic and admitted on a Tuesday to the Maternity Special Unity. She suffered from severe High blood pressure in pregnancy. Her baby died in her womb, while at home, owing to this high blood pressure. Her pregnancy was only 25 weeks calculated by Ultra Sound Scan.

My firm was the last team of Doctors to care for her. Four teams had attended to her since admission.

'On Call' meant that a team of ten or so Doctors worked 24hrs in Maternity and Gynecology Emergency wards. There were five teams, called firms, in the Department. Each firm was headed by two or more Consultants. This meant that the hospital operated 24/7 at the highest level of care in the country.

Change of shift or 'Hand Over' took place at 0730 and was characterized by rigorous screening of all patients the incoming firm was inheriting. Any one patient the incoming firm thought had been miss managed, called for serious explanations by the outgoing firm. This done, a new treatment plan, agreed upon by the consultants of the two firms, would be put in place.

These hand over rounds also served as an internal Audit in the department on the level of care being offered to the patients. Junior Doctors were expected to present patients to consultants and any Doctor found to be lacking in Knowledge was instantly lambasted. The faint hearted cried during these rounds. Any Doctor lacking in knowledge hated the hand over round. It was not uncommon for a fight to erupt during these rounds.

The knowledge expected at post graduate level was even higher. The answers and information demanded by some consultants made medicine as tough as rocket science at NASA. What they had learnt in twenty years of practice, you had to learn in just a couple of months.

I was a first year post graduate student, with five years working experience. In this department, my work experience counted for nothing. As far as my consultants were concerned, I was a mere first year Post graduate student, however on this day, I would present a paradigm shift.

During her four days stay in hospital, Mulenga must have listened attentively to the case presentations of her illness over and over again. The debates that raged around her must have perplexed and overwhelmed her.

Doctors' handover took place on patients' bed side. I am sure the information that came out of these rounds was quickly relayed to state house.

Clinically she was quite ill, temperature raised to 39 degrees centigrade. I could only think of sepsis. Malaria was highly unlikely. I feared she might have a ruptured uterus.

The order in the file was to increase her dose of medicine to enable her expel the dead baby via the birth canal.

I examined her abdomen thoroughly and was suddenly brought to a halt by my strange findings.

I immediately pulled my phone, leaned against the side window and called my senior colleague;

"Doc, did you examine this patient?" I started. "I think the baby is not in the womb. This is a ruptured uterus. She will need an immediate operation. This temperature is not due to malaria. It is infection from the dead baby in the belly. There is pus in this abdomen."

"Are you sure doc?" he answered with doubt in his voice. "If that's what you think, please go ahead. I am out of the hospital for supper."

"I think this womb tore more than two days ago,' I concluded.

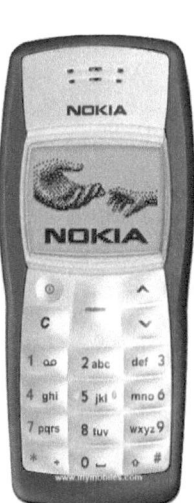

I hardly put down my faithful Nokia Eleven Hundred than the 'bedsider' handed me her gold plated *iphone*.

"Who are you?" The voice on the other end demanded angrily. "All the senior Doctors have told me that she must be delivered the normal way because the baby is dead."

I cut the phone without answering and turned to the woman.

"Who was that?" I demanded.

"That was her father. He is a Minister at State House and is the brother to the president," She answered triumphantly.

"What?" I asked. I thought I heard Mafia at state house.

It was at this point that I learnt about her VIP status.

"Why didn't someone warn me about Princess Fiona here?" I thought to myself.

Had I known who she was, I probably wouldn't have exposed her abdomen let alone touched it for examination. I would have simply followed what was written on her file. After all, she had been seen by the best. Who needs a first year student, when you are a VIP?

Had she died, the pathologist conducting the postmortem would have probably written the following words; 'cause of death; Obstetrical Negligence. Now negligence is a failure to exercise the care that a reasonably prudent person would exercise in like circumstances

While I was still recollecting my thoughts, the patient pulled her phone and called her husband.

Within seconds, he zoomed in like a Genie ejecting out of a magic lamp.

"Please save my wife Doc, these people have turned her into a political yoyo," he started to explain, his huge body trembling. "If you are sure of what you are saying, please go ahead and operate. Give me the consent form, I will sign it."

Mulenga looked at me with begging eyes to proceed as her husband had said. She didn't say any words but her silence said it all. She was only 26years old and about to place her life in a total stranger's hands.

Standing there brought me vivid memories of another incredible patient I had looked after six months earlier. She too had been on this same bed, suffering from severe hypertension in pregnancy. She was called Mrs. Subra.

Once the consent was signed, I hurried to theatre. I hardly left labor ward than my eleven hundred rang again. You guessed right, it was the voice of the angry Minister hurling commands at me.

"I have talked to the director of the Hospital, the head of department and the president has been informed, do not touch that patient. We are going to fly her to South Africa on Monday for specialist treatment," He commanded.

I was outraged when I heard this non medical directive. I was not going to get instructions from any politician that had no respect for Local Specialists and totally ignorant about medical Emergencies. This was an emergency and all he cared about was a fancy ride to RSA. The patient was too ill to wait for Monday and let alone survive the flight to RSA. It was now State decision vs Medical decision, a very difficult decision to be faced with.

Mulenga's caring husband had already mandated me to help save his wife. And that's what I was going to do. My colleagues and I had vowed to pursue the fifth millennium Development Goal in our own version. We called it 'Zero Tolerance to Maternal Death'. I considered making a call to my consultant, but couldn't tell how many were muzzled by the state machinery. A political directive to evacuate her would have scared many a consultant. Besides, her womb had burst open under their noses.

I got to the change room in theatre and begun to think, "A dim witted Doctor in the state machinery, would have been pleased to accompany the patient and amuse himself at the prospects of shopping in RSA from his travel allowances."

I wondered how the referral letter to Morning side clinic would have been worded. I was sure the letter would have read something like this;

"To the Specialists at Morning side Hospital, We refer to you the President's Niece for further Specialist evaluation. All our doctors are in the opposition."

"She can easily die on you in theatre and you would be blacklisted, ending your medical career," a strange voice in my mind cautioned me.

"This isn't a matter of heroism, this patient needs immediate surgical intervention," I reminded the voice.

She was brought in the operating theatre and within minutes the operation was under way at 21:45.

Once inside the abdominal cavity, I was able to examine the full extent of her dire condition. The baby lay in mire of pus and exudative fluid on the mother's intestines. The uterus had ruptured longitudinally emptying its contents into the abdominal cavity. I picked the dead baby still attached to its placenta and handed it to the mid wife. I then turned my attention to the soiling in the abdomen and set out to wash Mulenga's internal organs copiously with saline. Satisfied with the wash out, I proceeded to close her surgical wound and sent her to the ward.

The angry minister called 15 minutes after I left theatre. This time, I summoned all my cranial nerves and fought back. I made him listen. I begun to explain the findings but he cut the phone.

Had I allowed the minister's daughter to wait until Monday, she would have died from infection and multiple organ failure.

The following day I went to review Mulenga on the ward, but found her file had gone missing. I later learnt it had actually been stolen.

All I could think about at that point was the agony of shifting anxiously waiting for me. I took a photo and headed for my old home to begin the search for new accommodation.

'A little picture is worth a thousand words'; I recited a Chinese proverb and left still in my scrubs.

I expected to be called to answer questions over the decision I had taken over the President's niece and even face suspension pending investigations. I feared the long arm of the law would soon visit me.

So I decided to visit my barber shop to *shave* my head in potato cut style as a sign of protest against political interference and wore a suite for work that gave me a Zuma look. I was feeling like a free statesman of Cape Town.

I was ready for war.

However none came. No one called me, not even the angry minister.

Politics had interfered with the care of this young lady right from the start.

Her husband confirmed this when he said, "Doc, these people have turned my wife into a political yoyo. I am not even allowed to make any decisions over my own wife."

I was now certain all the Doctors that saw her earlier in the week erred in their judgment because of political interference.

They had pushed attempts for a vaginal birth too far resulting into a uterine rupture, severe sepsis and nearly ending into a fatality.

Mulenga stayed on the ward for six days and was then discharged from hospital free of complications within a week.

Three months went by and I had by now forgotten about saving the extended first family however the long arm of the law hadn't. It caught up with me one afternoon in the hospital car park. The court messenger was the hospital managing director.

"Good afternoon doc," came a greeting from a familiar gruff voice through my car window.

"Good afternoon sir," I answered.

"There is something you did and my office has received a huge sum of money for it. I have been instructed to inform you that you must find accommodation in Lusaka at whatever cost and the source will pay for it," he explained sitting down in the passenger's seat.

"I certainly need accommodation," I answered studying his body language carefully. "However, I am not aware of a service in which I asked for inducement or obtained recompense."

"It's state house and that's all you should know," he stated with a queer smile.

"It's about the president niece. I know you heard. I disobeyed the president. I am sure I will be dismissed from your hospital," I answered smiling as I reflected on the night of this difficult decision with nostalgia. "Did you read her file? It went missing. I hope it made it to your office intact."

"Actually, you saved the president's niece and because of you, he is very proud of Zambian doctors that make a difference like you have done. He wants to meet you. I am very proud of you too. I saw the file; excellent work doc. Now go on, run get yourself a five star house in Lusaka," he spoke with true admiration of my complex decision I faced.

It would take four years before our paths would cross again. Mulenga was expecting.

The couple caught up with me at a rural hospital where I was stationed and requested me to be their Doctor. I was so glad to see this wonderful couple again. I reflected on our first encounter and breathed a sigh of relief.

They met me recovering from the first phase of shock; from the tragedy that befell me. My House Burnt to Ashes in broad day light around 1pm. The inferno devoured a decade of the labors of my hands. Nothing was recovered from the House. Twenty one days had passed since.

When I saw this couple that morning, it made me rethink my loss. Their loss dwarfed my own infinitely. This was Mulenga's fifth pregnancy but had lost all her previous unborn babies to a severe form of High Blood Pressure peculiar to pregnancy.

They handed me the medical file containing my surgical notes of the operation I had performed on Mulenga four years previously. I read these notes filled with nostalgia of my time at the University Hospital and the night her husband and I were faced with the difficulty decision to go ahead and operate amidst Political calls to evacuate Mulenga to South Africa. Her husband was no ordinary man; he took charge of the desperate situation and made the brave decision to sign the consent for the Emergency Surgery to save his wife. I could only imagine the burning reproach and chastisement he may have received from his in-laws. Many in his shoes would have opted to fly to South Africa, carrying a frail wife, and ending up losing their beloved spouse.

That morning, I sketched out the medical voyage Mulenga would sail in this precarious pregnancy as seen by my human eyes. This was a journey requiring the Almighty Hand of God. It was beyond ordinary Medical Science. **It would take a Miracle to see her through.**

In His Hands

The year is June 2007. She lay on her sick bed crying, "I want my baby, I want my baby, I want my baby….," she had no one willing to hear her plea.

The decision had been made at the top and it was final. The senior doctors made this decision.

I had recently joined a residence program to pursue a master's degree in obstetrics and gynecology. My firm took calls on Friday. There were five firms in all. We were the last team in a weekly call schedule and shared weekend calls in the Department of Obstetrics and Gynecology of the University Hospital.

I met Yumbe on one such grilling Friday calls. This particular one had been very busy. There were far too many very ill mothers admitted to our special observation units and Annex in labor ward. Majority of these mothers had pregnancies complicated by high blood pressure. They had suffered convulsions in pregnancy, a disease referred to as Eclampsia.

Yumbe was one such patient who was gravely ill. She was swollen all over the body. Her face was brutally distorted and could not manage to open her eyes. She had been admitted on a Sunday, five days before our firm took call. That meant she had been handed down from firm to firm and cared for by the highest expertise in the Department, the consultants of Obstetrics and Gynecology. The department and firms were run like military Units. The consultants issued the commands and we the postgraduate students carried them out.

The command had been issued to terminate Yumbe's pregnancy. The phrase 'patient has not yet expelled' echoed throughout her file, page after page since the day she was admitted.

It would take five days plus one awkward hour, in the early hours of a freezing June Saturday morning before I met her. This was to be an incredible encounter in my line of duty.

I reported for work as I always did but was late for the hand over round. Meaning, I never got to learn about this sick mother. I went straight to theatre.

Our firm was headed by two wonderful consultants. Under them were three postgraduate (PGs) students at fourth, third and first year level respectively. I was in first. Below me were several junior resident medical officers. Below the junior doctors were several seventh and fifth year medical students. Together we formed a formidable team referred to us firm E.

Theatre was extremely busy on this call day. Usually the postgraduates took turns in theatre. We attended to Emergency cases needing surgical intervention as well as teaching Junior doctors Surgery, particularly Caesarean Sections.

Before enrolling onto the master's program, I worked at a busy mission Hospital where I learnt basic general surgery to advanced bowel surgery that involved resection and stitching intestines.

I was also privileged to work under various specialists visiting our mission hospital. I learnt advanced operations on the womb.

I was also thoroughly taught, removal of the uterus (Hysterectomy) in emergencies complete with its cervix. Owing to this background, I possessed greater surgical training among the junior postgraduate students. At eight minutes operating time, personal record, for normal caesarean sections, I was among the fastest surgeons in the Department. And a theatre favorite among anesthetists and theatre nurses on busy days.

I was so busy in theatre on this call day that I never saw the sun set. I left theatre at 8pm for 'Lunch'. The final year postgraduate student took over theatre from me. She was to cover till midnight. The hours from midnight to 4am were covered by the third year student. I would be back in theatre from 4am till handover time at 8am. Coverage meant you were responsible for the labor ward and gynecological Emergency wards, supervising the junior members of the team and answering to consultations.

With the time table agreed among us, I drove off the hospital to a fast food cafe in Kabulonga.

After my late lunch, I headed straight to the post graduate call room. I had some reading to catch up on, but was too tired to get anything past my eyes. So I decided I had had enough for the day and retired to catch some sleep. I gave my watch one look, and like a traffic officer at rush hour, it pointed harshly to two hours past midnight.

I was woken up by a sound I thought was a call from labor ward. I checked my beeper, checked my phone, there were no missed calls. It was three in the morning and it was freezing outside. I checked my colleague's bed; his beddings had not been touched. He was still in the operating theatre.

I tried to return to sleep, but was overcome by a feeling that there was a patient urgently needing my attention in labor ward. I decided to call labor ward immediately. The midwife who answered my call reassured me it was quiet in labor ward and that I could continue with my rest. However I failed find rest despite this assurance from the midwife. I decided to check on the critically ill mothers in Annex.

No sooner had I entered Annex than I heard these words; 'I want my baby, I want my baby'... she sobbed uncontrollably between these words. All my attention was now drawn to this one patient...

"I wonder why she is crying," I thought to myself. The obvious thought that came to my mind was the exact one you would have thought had you had been in my shoes at that early hour. "Has she lost her baby?" Mothers in this room were luck to survive eclampsia, let alone their babies. This disease was notoriously responsible for more still births than any I could think of at that moment. It would be fifteen minutes before I talked with her.

She was surrounded by a blanket of relatives, praying earnestly for her. They hardly gave any notice to me standing there. I decided I would wait, for these were no ordinary prayers exploding from the room. It also gave me the time to quickly peruse through her file.

I learnt from the file, this was her 6th day since admission for severe pre eclampsia. Literately, that is to say for a disease unique to pregnancy before the mother starts convulsing. The disease had damaged her kidneys, liver and the clotting system.

The brain was showing signs that she would seizure at any moment. It was very clear this was a critically ill mother. The solemn faces of the intercessors about her bed plainly reflected her calamitous condition.

24year old Yumbe had recently married and was trying to have her first born child.

In the natural this wasn't going to happen. The situation called for a 'Foolish decision'. After all, the ways of God are foolish to the learned. With maternal mortality at 830 at national level, no woman should die giving life. It was ok for the baby to die in order to save the mother. However, it wasn't going to be this baby; Yumbe's baby would live.

"I want my baby, I want my baby, I want my baby," the cries continued echoing from her bed.

When I finally got my turn, I approached her bed, introduced myself and requested to examine her. The pregnancy barely went past her umbilicus. By her dates she was 32 weeks pregnant. Physical examination placed the pregnancy at less than 24 weeks. It's no wonder the learned consultants were treating her pregnancy as an abortion.

Four firms saw her in the course of the week. Twice by the firm that admitted her. She had received several doses of medicines used to terminate a pregnancy. But she didn't expel despite the dose of the abortion drug being increased since admission. This gave rise to the phrase, 'patient has not expelled' page after page.

Despite claiming to be eight months pregnant, it was what the doctors saw that counted? A first time mother is more likely to error on her dates and so her dates are considered unreliable.

There was another explanation to this small pregnancy that the doctors conveniently ignored. It was possible Yumbe was truly eight months pregnant however her baby had failed to grow inside her womb owing to the high blood pressure she had suffered. A condition referred to as intra uterine growth restriction or IUGR. In which case, the safest mode of delivery for such a small and fragile infant would have been by caesarean section. However that would entail placing the mother's life at risk for a baby that would not survive life in a third world neonate unit. This delivery needed Gods intervention. Medical science was still in its infancy on this matter in this part of the world... Standing there, I asked myself numerous ethical questions;

"Is this a leave alone matter or is this a Linda rescue mission?"

I understood clearly what I was required to do medically. I was expected to increase the aborting dose and have her Expel. However, there was a new consultant at work now. The author of life himself, the Ancient of days; I could almost ascertain the Mysterious Call I heard was from him.

In medicine, however, such thoughts may be considered auditory hallucinations and necessitate a psychiatric evaluation. I could have been so tired and stressed that I was now beginning to Hear Voices. Conversely, anyone who has a father and has lived with his father knows his father's voice. Therefore it could also be argued that those who disobeyed their parents were juvenile delinquents. I was a child of God and I was always cognizant of that. Unfortunately, many of God's children today spit in his face and deny him vehemently. They have become a brood of vipers, a league of delinquents the world has ever seen since its creation.

"Ms Yumbe," I started to talk, "have the Doctors explained your condition?"

"Yes Doctor," she answered. "However I want my baby."

She sobbed as she had done probably since admission.

At this point, I requested to see her relatives and her husband. I wanted to be sure they all understood the decision that had been made. Working at University Hospital made me realize how bad at communication Doctors were. Fortunately, the whole family understood the danger Ms Yumbe was in and the efforts the doctors were making to save her life. I told them about all the risks the surgical option carried.

Like Yumbe, the whole family wanted her to have the baby. After all, this was medicine in the 21st century. It was expected to deliver a palatable solution to this precarious predicament; one acceptable by this desperate family. This meant, 'A live baby and a live mother', nothing less.

That clarified, I made a call to theatre informing them about this mother. With one voice, they said I could take her. This answer frightened me! I obviously expected a big NO! Especially that they had worked the whole night. And I was suggesting taking them a very ill mother who could easily die on the operating table. This would result in incident report writing, the last thing an exhausted theatre crew would want to find themselves in.

I had to find words for a quick short prayer. 'LORD, you have heard your daughter's prayer.' I stated briefly. Then I recited Jeremiah 1:5, "before I formed you in your mother's womb, I knew you".

That said, I headed for the operating theatre. The operation took only 11minutes. Delivery time was less than a minute. It was a male baby weighing 1.1kg. Vigorously kicking and crying. The baby was sent to our third world neonatal ward were babies this size rarely made it out alive. The mother was sent back to Annex. As for me, I hit the road and headed straight home. I chose to skip the handover round because no one was going to understand my decisions. It was a grave offence to change a consultant's decision, worse still a collective decision by them. One consultant once remarked, 'patients belonged to consultants only'.

I later learnt my colleagues were at pains to explain the decision I took. I returned to work on Monday expecting to be 'court marshaled'. No one raised the mater. Ms Yumbe made quick recovery and was fully ambulant by the second day. She was moved to the postnatal ward by second day of the operation.

I made every effort <u>NOT</u> to see her or her baby. I knew this had nothing to do with me and so I avoided any attention that could confer personal glory on me.

All glory belongs to God. I was simply a vessel handpicked to execute this 'foolish and dangerous decision'.

Two weeks went by before I ran into Ms Yumbe again. She was returning from the Neonatal ward to check on her miniature son.

"Doctor!" she exclaimed when she ran into me. "You don't come to see us, why?"

"I am happy to see you Ms Yumbe," I fumbled for words. "How are you? How is the baby?" I added quickly avoiding her question.

"The baby is fine but has lost weight," she answered. "He weighed 980g this morning."

I felt strength leave me. Our baby was now less than a kilo. That was going to be a tough battle in human terms. However this was no ordinary baby, neither was the mom. From that day on, I made it my mission to avoid running into Ms Yumbe at all costs.

It would be nine months before I ran into Ms Yumbe again. I bumped into her and her husband, on a Sunday, in a shopping mall, Shoprite

Manda Hill in Lusaka.

On seeing me, she flew over to where I stood and handed me the biggest baby I have ever seen. The shoppers stopped and stared in utter amusement. Her Indian Husband hurriedly chased behind her.

"This is your baby," she said. "We are from dedicating him to the LORD at bread of life church."

I looked to heaven and murmured, "thank you Father."

Nine months earlier, I held this baby on the palm of my hand but now I could hardly support him on my two outstretched arms.

I recalled how I had been woken up from my sleep by a Mysterious Call thinking it was a call from labor ward.

I could only sum it up in an old hymn and a fairy tale cliché;

"He's got the tiny Little Baby in His Hands

"All is well that ends well"

***

He's got the whole world in His hands
He's got the whole world in His hands
He's got the whole world in His hands
He's got the whole world in His hands

He's got the wind and the rain in His hands
He's got the wind and the rain in His hands
He's got the wind and the rain in His hands
He's got the whole world in His hands

He's got the tiny little baby in His hands
He's got the tiny little baby in His hands
He's got the tiny little baby in His hands
He's got the whole world in His hands

He's got you and me, brother, in His hands,

He's got you and me, brother, in His hands,

He's got you and me, brother, in His hands,

He's got the whole world in His hands.

He's got you and me sister, in His hands

He's got you and me sister, in His hands

He's got you and me sister, in His hands

He's got the whole world in His hands

He's got ev'rybody here in His hands.

He's got ev'rybody here in His hands.

He's got ev'rybody here in His hands.

He's got the whole world in His hands.

LUSHUPO

Three weeks earlier, I was posted to work at a mission hospital in chief Macha's chiefdom. The hospital was located 75km from the nearest town of Choma and a Grade C category under the Dutch Rural Retention Scheme for Doctors. This meant a hard to reach area. 'I marched, like a Knight, carrying his weapon ready for war...'

***

"Oxcart injuries are as ghastly as Road traffic Accidents", I thought to myself after concluding a thorough abdominal examination on a twelve year old boy brought to our Emergency Room. His abdomen was grossly distended suggestive of internal bleeding. The Bleeding was caused by injury to his Spleen. 24hrs had elapsed since the accident.

It was harvest time in the village and excitement echoed across the chiefdom. At last their toil and sweat had come to fruition. They had a bumper harvest.

However for Lushupo's family, their excitement was to be disrupted by a tragic accident.

The boys in this village were responsible for bringing in the harvest from the fields using 0xe driven carts. In order to meet the daily tonnage goals, they drove these carts with ferocity like Roman soldiers in their chariots.

Watching at a distance gave you a feeling of time travel, far into the distant past when oxen and horses ruled the road, to a time when horses were Ferraris and carts limousines.

Three weeks earlier, I had been posted to work at a mission hospital in chief Macha's chiefdom. The hospital was located 75km from the nearest town of Choma and a Grade C category under the Dutch Rural Retention Scheme for Doctors. This meant a hard to reach area. There were three other Doctors at the station; unfortunately none had assisted later on operated on a ruptured spleen. I was the junior most of the team, comprising two board certified family practitioners and a senior General Practitioner.

At this hospital, the ER served as consultation room as well; and was shared by three doctors seated at 12 O'clock, 3 O'clock and 7 O'clock in this six by four centimeter haunted room. The information desk at 2 O'clock added to the chaos of the already crowded ER. The staff at the hospital called this place simply as Room 13. It was a place where anything, including ghosts and demons could come knocking at the door.

When Lushupo came knocking in Room 13, the obvious thing was to refer this boy to the nearby district hospital which had a surgeon. The Journey would take three to four hours on a treacherous gravel road. Lushupo was admitted to male surgical ward pending referral for surgery.

Before transport could be arranged, we were called back to the ward by the nurse on duty. She couldn't read his blood pressure. It had become unrecordable.

We immediately knew what this meant. The boy was losing blood at supersonic speed and unless a miracle, he was going to die. He wouldn't make it to the District Hospital. The patient had gone into hemorrhagic shock.

Prior to my posting to Macha, I worked at Ndola Central Hospital on the copper belt province. My rotation in department of surgery was the most exciting time I spent at this hospital. It was known to my seniors that my calls were synonymous with a ruptured spleen. I do not recall a single call day when I didn't diagnose a ruptured spleen in the emergency room however I could not be allowed to operate for I was too junior and the patients critically ill for a novice in surgery.

I watched each operation curiously in theatre and on occasions was allowed a place as second assistant on the operation table. I had recently graduated from Medical school with a bachelor's degree in Surgery and Medicine. Three months had passed since arriving at the famous Ndola central hospital for my internship.

Watching that boy deteriorate while we stood helplessly that afternoon brought back memories of the Casualty department at Ndola Central Hospital. The leading causes of injury were Road Traffic Accidents.

Here I was, deep in a rural hospital, confronted with an oxcart injury that was as grisly as a motor vehicle accident.

I couldn't stand watch Lushupo die. And so I told the other doctors I could operate if they would let me try.

"Have you ever operated on a spleen injury before?" one doctor asked me. "Suppose you find the liver and mesentery injured, what will you do?"

"No," I answered. "However I have assisted in this sort of surgery before."

There was a long silence as they pondered over my offer. The ultra sound had suggested splenic injury only. I was fully aware of the possibilities of finding additional injuries.

"If we do nothing and waste time standing like a bunch of corrupt Judges he will definitely die," I said breaking the silence. "It's better; I kill him in theatre trying to save his life."

Reluctantly, they agreed I could try.

Having squeezed out permission to operate, I was confronted with yet another major problem; the hospital did not have an Anesthetist let alone an Anesthesiologist.

The anesthesia to be used was as critical as the operation to be done. The only crude aesthetic cocktail the other Doctors could give was a drug called ketamin. This preparation, generally not suitable for this type of operation, works by sending a patient into a deep sleep, into a state referred to as dissociative amnesia. However, the patient would be able to breathe own his own. This means, once you open the abdomen, intestines pop up out of the abdominal cavity obscuring your way to the site of injury.

Furthermore, ketamine does not relax the muscles of the abdomen making surgery very difficult

The task ahead now seamed a 'No win situation'. "Should I back off and let the boy die?"' I thought to myself. I had never seen this operation done under this drug. Neither had I seen it done in a child this age.

I recalled the words of a professor of anatomy in medical school while dissecting a region of the abdomen I was about to enter in this operation.

He said, "a blind man can operate on a spleen that ruptures in its capsule."

These words were a riddle to me at the time. What he meant was; provided the capsule is not breached, you don't have to operate at all. The capsule acts like a seal, preventing continued bleeding.

"You see class," Prof. would say when stating a matter of clinical importance. "The spleen receives its blood supply from a large blood vessel called the splenic artery. It shares a source of blood as the liver and the stomach. This means a lot of blood indeed. The splenic artery runs a predictable course, passing under the stomach to the spleen on the left side of the body. Here, the spleen is closely related to the; left kidney, the tail of the pancreas, the stomach and the colon. If one passed his hand just adjacent to the greater curvature of the stomach and pressed down towards the back, he would feel a pulse of a large vessel. This is the splenic artery. When the spleen is injured and its capsule remains intact, the patient can be monitored conservatively. Look out for his blood pressure and pulse. This is known as expectant management. Don't go out pulling out all spleens that get injured. Some of your patients will need their spleens, especially the young. You don't need eyes to see this.

I took my position at the operating table and as was the custom at this hospital, we offered a prayer for guidance. Soon the operation was under way. The theatre nurse handed me a scalpel and without hesitation I proceeded to make an incision from the bottom of his breast bone down to his navel. As soon as I passed the muscles, a dark looking zone propped up in my view. It was like peering down a deep haunted sea. "Heamoperi toneum!" I exclaimed to myself.

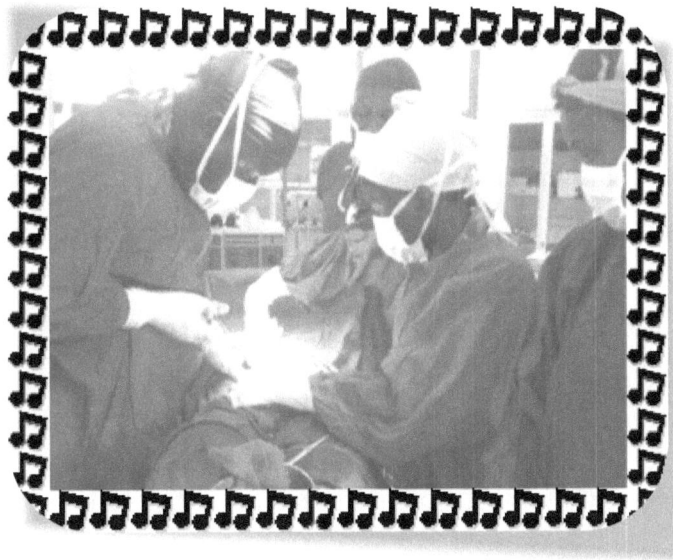

This was the last I could see, from here downward; I entered professor's proverbial blind fold surgery. I worked my hand towards the territory of the ghost artery with my heart pounding heavily as if it was last minute penalty shootout in a final football match.

Theatre was dead silent; you could hear the thoughts of all the doctors in the room. I worked enjoying the silence to the sound of Mozart's Classics playing deep in the Limbic System of my brain.

"I have found it!" I announced victoriously. The others didn't join in to celebrate my discovery.

"I have the splenic artery," I said plainly.

There was a sigh of relief in theatre. I placed clumps on the bleeding artery and ligated it.

The spleen itself had suffered a burst injury ending up in multiple fragments till its holding capsule begun to give way. It was this capsule that made it possible for the boy to reach the hospital but now it could no longer prevent the continued bleeding.

I cleaned the abdomen of the blood that had   accumulated from internal bleeding, revealing a wonder of God. This boy had extra spleens, a feature known as ectopic spleen. This thrilled the other Doctors and one quickly scrubbed in to touch this amazing feature.

"He didn't need his spleen after all, he had plenty to spare," I thought to myself.

Removal of the spleen would have placed the patient at great risk to infection caused by a particular strain of Germs known as encapsulated bacteria.

The rest of the surgery proceeded without incidence. The wounded spleen was removed complete and care taken not to injure the tail of his pancreas.

Lushupo stayed in hospital for seven days and made incredible recovery beyond everyone's expectations. He was eating his regular diet by third day post surgery.

At discharge his family allowed me to change his name to Lushomo, meaning Faith. His old name, Lushupo, had a connotation of being a difficult and troublesome boy. Had he been a girl, Linda, would have been my choice of names.

This was among the first of the major decisions and surgeries I would be faced with in my practice of medicine. The days that followed gave me a feeling of surgical triumph and a sense of awe to God. Was this a freak act of lucky, or an act of surgical genius or a miracle of God? I chose to believe the later.

9-1-1

I met David at the height of my War at home and at Work. I was on 28 days urgent affairs leave from work without any intention of ever returning.

My mind had been made up to leave following a scuffle with my supervisor. She misinterpreted my late coming on one busy call day to be absconding work. She went on to write a misguided letter and copied it to heads of departments and hospital director. She stated in her letter that I had taken my accommodation hitch to be more important than my CALL day. I considered her letter totally misguided, unfortunate and utter baloney.

Meanwhile at home, my delectable spouse accused me bitterly of placing my work above her. She complained that I was always studying and not spending time at home but with patients at the hospital.

She obviously didn't understand what Post graduate training demanded no matter how much I tried to explain. She, instead, was preoccupied with family expansion at the time and was expecting our second child. Fortunately the new arrival turned out to be a fine dolly baby boy.

For the first time I found myself agreeing with the Author of a book entitled 'Internship' I had read. He had argued, in his book, that internship was not a time to run off to the mountains to get married and have children but rather a time when the study of medicine really begun. I read this book in my first year of University and at the time, it didn't make sense at all. No one in their right frame of mind would spend seven years studying medicine only to be told the true study of medicine begun in your eighth year... "What manner of a career is this where after seven long gruesome years of study; you were still considered too ignorant to work without supervision." The seven years in medical school served only as an introduction to the complex Art and Science of Medicine. The pressure on my mind had reached atomic fission proportions and equaled several Fukushima and Chernobyl combined. A melt down was looming on the horizon.

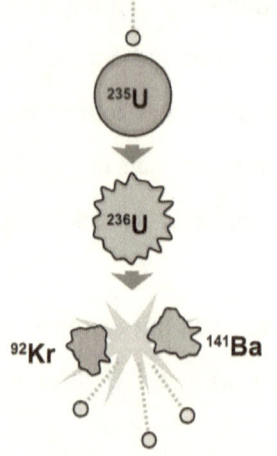

Going by the author of that book, marriage was getting in the way of my pursuit of a Master's degree in Medicine. The pressure I experienced was palpable even to the novice. I depressurized by busying myself at the office.

I ran a consultation office in town to try my hand at private practice. I called my practice Caring Cross. With my books locked away and no calls to look forward to, I started my days' routine at ease.

One cold Lusaka Wednesday morning, I decided to visit a shopping mall in order to stock up on my dwindling office stationary supplies. I drove down to Manda hill in heavy traffic, only to change my mind once in the store.

I found myself wandering to the electronic section of Game stores. Realizing my planned shopping had turned into an aimless stroll, I left the Mall without buying anything. I was happy to leave and proud not to have made an impetuous purchase. I turned my Landcruiser VX into Great East road and drove into city center. Traffic was heavy towards Northmead shopping complex. Several Taxi drivers hooted incessantly at the slow moving vehicles at the front. They drove their blue min buses carelessly, displaying typical Lusaka hooliganism and broke every written traffic rule.

Back at the office, I tried to concentrate on some creative thinking but realized I had run out of the materials to use. These could only be bought from Game at Manda hill. This was the same shopping complex I had walked away from that morning. It took about an hour and half to drive from my office in heavy Lusaka traffic to the mall.

Once at Manda Hill, I rushed into Game and headed straight for the stationary section.

I stared bluntly at the laminating paper I wanted. On seeing the obese price tag, I changed my mind again. I didn't need this paper after all; I comforted myself as I walked away from this section. I decided to wonder about once again in the shop. I moved from section to section even the candy section and I picked myself some chocolates to nibble in traffic.

At this point I realized I was being drawn to this store to find someone. I was well familiar with this feeling ever since I met Linda at Mpelembe

Secondary School. Happening in a shopping mall was a bit odd to me. These déjà vu encounters have happened to me in the hospital numerous times but never in a shop. So I decided to leave, convinced I was being a psychic freak. I don't believe in clairvoyant phenomenon. I believe God speaks to us in strange ways. I had the sense to know if this was God, he would make it clear at the appropriate moment in time. So, I hurried out of the shop into the car park and drove off for my office. I hardly sat at my desk than the phone rang.

"This is Pill of health," the voice on the other end explained. "We have a cheque for you and you need to collect it today."

"Whose cheque is it for?" I asked. "I am sure you called a wrong number. Check your details. You don't owe me any money."

"A Cheque of $9000," my heart missed a beat when she read the dollar value. "Doc, come collect your money."

"I am coming right away," I fumbled for my car keys and hastily reached for the door.

"Sir, you have a client," Sepiso my faithful receptionist ran after me.

"Reschedule her appointment," I called back.

"But Doc...," Sepiso tried to explain something.

"Hold the Lift," I called after the lady in the Lift. My office was on the 7th floor of Kulima Tower building.

I did locum at this private clinic the previous year and had since given my clinic away to a friend. There was no way I would be owed money by this prosperous private hospital.

I was interested to verify this anomaly. The cheque turned out to be real and a generous sum was engraved across its face. It was enough to please any broke fellow in my shoes. I grabbed the cheque and departed the premises for the nearest bank at Manda Hill.

To this day, I am not sure I understood what I was being paid for. However I had been too broke to raise audit questions.

With the cheque secured in my breast pocket, I found myself fighting the urge to head for the stationery shop at Manda Hill Shopping Mall. Suddenly, I found the obese price tags on the stationary I wanted extremely lean. I headed straight for the bank first. With the money safely in the bank, I set out to do some window shopping. As you would guess, I went back to my rendezvous Store, cautious this time, I had to find someone.

I decided, instead, to let them find me and so I walked slowly from section to section on tenterhooks. This search brought me many memorable moments of childhood when we played hide and seek with the neighbors' dimwitted kids and a pretty girl next door. In my childhood, there was always a pretty girl next door.

David was one of the workers in this magnificent shopping mall. He was a marketing supervisor and someone I went to high school with. Sixteen years had gone by since.

I often met David whenever I was in this store. And so when he saw me that morning, he came by to say hello as he always did when I visited. We chatted briefly about old times and touched on current affairs. He asked me to see him when I was done with my shopping and strode away. I couldn't tell him that I was responding to a 911 call right inside his shop. I was now shopping for a person I had no clue they even existed. I never told anyone these strange extrasensory insights. It was a gift which was best kept to one self. It had served me well in my school days. I often knew the topics we would be examined on.

I walked around all the sections of the shop, including those I hardly entered. I found myself entering the camping and fishing section however the mysterious person remained elusive. I gave the shop one final sweep but still there was no sight of the mystery man or woman. I prepared to leave glad it had been a false alarm. Deep down my heart I knew the search wasn't over yet.

I went to see David on my way out of the store. He wanted to know how I spent my Lusaka weekends as he saw me to the exit.

"So where are you found nowadays," he asked as we reached the exit.

"I run a pass time maternity house Call Clinic in Makeni," I answered.

"Really," he remarked surprised. "My wife is pregnant at home and her blood pressure was high at the clinic yesterday."

On hearing this, I knew immediately David was the 911 call. The cheque from Pill of health was God's way to get me back to Manda hill and to David.

"So it is you who dialed 911," I stopped and gave him a puzzling gaze.

"I don't understand," David looked visibly confused.

"Take me to see your wife at once," I commanded him.

He got urgent permission to leave work and in the twinkling of an eye we were headed for his house.

On the way, he narrated to me how he and his wife have lost four babies in the womb to hypertension. This was the wife's fifth pregnancy and was worried a similar thing was going to happen.

Their only child was aged nine. His wife was due the previous week and had been seen at University Hospital with raised blood pressure. Unfortunately, she was told to return in a week for review.

"The doctor who advised this was insane and an assassin," I thought to myself.

That morning she had gone to the clinic because of a headache, blurring of vision and swelling of legs.

Once at the house, I asked for her antenatal card and found the BP at the clinic was 190/130. And she was now 42 weeks by her dates, meaning she should have delivered a week before last. This baby had matured in her womb four weeks previously and could even have been delivered then.

The pregnancy itself looked as though she was carrying twins. She needed an urgent delivery or there was a high risk they would lose this baby too. The tribulations facing this baby were enormous; High Blood Pressure, overweight referred to as fetal Macrosomia, over stay in the womb or post dates and previous loss of this baby's unborn siblings.

A tsunami was raging in this womb and the Call to evacuate the womb was long overdue. It was only by God that this baby was still holding on. High Risk Pregnancy has an unsavory notoriety; there is a tendency of poor outcomes to repeat themselves.

"I am taking you to hospital right away," I told her in a firm but empathetic voice. "Your blood pressure is too high. You will need a caesarean delivery today."

She looked at her husband in disbelief and visibly wondered at the stranger her husband had brought to their house. After a brief audible silence, she asked to be allowed to take a bath.

"No, we have no time to waste. We must leave immediately," I protested.

We jumped into my Ambulance and headed straight for the hospital. I called a friend in the operating theatre and scheduled Mrs. David for surgery. My colleague planned to operate on her as soon as we were at the hospital.

While on the way to hospital, I explained the dangers of raised blood pressure in pregnancy to my stunned 9-1-1 patient.

"Hypertension in pregnancy can damage the brain, liver, kidneys and clotting system. The baby can die in the womb suddenly without warning. This disease is responsible for numerous maternal deaths in our country."

"How do you know it is a boy?" she asked confused.

"Honey, don't question God's angel," said David resting his hand on his wife's large waist.

"It will be a boy, you will see," I stole a glance at Mrs. David. It was clear this pregnancy had grotesquely rearranged her beauty. She wore a lovely white stole made out of fur which loosely covered her shoulders. This scarf or wrap greatly accentuated her new features.

David was a good man. He had not run away from home like most common men would in his shoes. He still returned home every evening to his large wife. I thought he too transformed into a gargantuan man eating Giant, the ugly green Ogre, when the Sun went down.

As these strange thoughts about Ogres raced in my sober mind, I guided the cruiser out of Addis Abba road to join Independence Avenue. We passed the High Court and Supreme Court magnificent buildings on our left. I wondered how the Honorable Judges would have handled this case if they were Obstetricians. I was certain the Judges would have granted the lawyers more time to study the evidence before arriving at a decision. They would have allowed length testimonies from all parties concerned. Lawyers representing the unborn infant would probably have acted as I, push for a speed delivery of justice.

Whereas lawyers representing the mother, would have probably pushed to delay the case and asked for time, measured in months, to prepare a catalogue of witnesses from the village.

We arrived at the hospital on a journey that seemed to have taken millennia.

Mrs. David was immediately wheeled into theatre. I remained with her husband to keep him calm but soon disappeared into theatre too. The caesarean was a success and she gave birth to a baby boy weighing 4.7kg. We were all thrilled by this good outcome.

We called this 9-1-1 Gift from heaven, 'Small Big Baby David Jr'. The boy was admitted to the neonatal unit because he was very big. Usually such big babies tend to be diabetic and have to be monitored closely before they can be allowed to go home. Mother and baby were discharged from hospital on day five in perfect health.

***

Here is my reflection on the above encounter

I think each day of our lives; God is looking for ordinary men and women to send to meet various needs. No matter how small that need may seem, God is pleased to meet it; to feed the hungry, visit the prisoners, cloth the naked, visiting the sick in hospital, looking after orphans and widows, etc

We don't have to feed the whole world or cloth the whole earth, or be aired on Television for all to see to gain his approval. Simply do to others what you would have them do to you. Where ever God sends you, he will also equip you with tools you will need to do his work.

It is, however, our human responsibility to learn these earthly tools. God has granted us abilities and understanding to attain their mastery. If you are a teacher, learn your subject; if you are a farmer, plant the seed; if you are a Judge, uphold justice; if you are a mathematician, know your numbers; if you are a nurse, take care of the sick without grumbling; if you are a Doctor, Practice your medicine with diligence; if you are an Engineer, master your Engineering; if you are a Banker, learn your banking; if you are a Manager, manage with wisdom; If you are a student, read your books diligently.

God will turn ordinary tools in our hands into extra ordinary tools for his service and that of our fellow man.

From a Drop of Water

I sat on my bed still thinking about Rhoda, a patient the hospital had set aside for me. By now, it was 8pm in Mbala. I decided to take a hot bathe to refresh my exhausted mind. Hardly five minutes into my cozy shower than my phone rang. It was the hospital.

"Dr Marximillian, this is the coverage nurse. I got your number from Dr Kalunda. We have just admitted a patient with suspected intestinal obstruction, a referral from Mpulungu hospital. The doctor on call is requesting for your opinion as there is no blood in the hospital," a male nurse, with a fun accent, explained.

"Send transport to pick me at Giza Inn. I am in room 12," I answered.

I dried myself quickly and dressed hurriedly. I had not had supper. And suddenly I felt very hungry. I quickly made myself coffee and opened a pack of biscuits as I let my mind wander at the worst case scenario awaiting me at the hospital; gangrenous compound sigmoid colon volvulus was top on my list together with a gangrenous ceacal volvulus. I was sure to be gone for a very long time if I was faced by any one of these killer afflictions.

The driver arrived shortly. We drove to the hospital in a landcruiser along the bumpy road Dr Kalunda and I had used earlier that day. I bounced up and down in the passenger seat. The empty chairs at the back rattled endlessly to the hospital.

I alighted at the entrance to the administration block and speeded for the operating theatre. The Doctor on call had decided to book the patient for immediate surgery and went back to his house to continue with his sleep.

I was met by the coverage nurse that had made the call. He was a serious looking young fellow whom I liked immediately. Several nurses and students were there to watch me stumble with my first major case at Abercorn.

I emerged from the male change room and hurriedly found my way through the maze of the colossal theatre. I deeply loved this Abercorn theatre. There was enough space for a dozen to play hide and seek. I found the patient, a young man in his early twenties, had already been placed on the operating table. He was in obvious distress and deeply jaundiced. I proceeded to examine the patient's abdomen. What I found surprised everyone.

"This patient has peritonitis," I announced to the anxious onlookers. "I will need a minimum of twelve litres of normal saline to wash his abdomen."

"We only have two litres of Ringer's lactate in theatre," the theatre nurse announced.

"Coverage, get me ten litres of saline before I wash your patient's abdomen with tap water," I answered. "Nurse, you can start scrubbing, I will join you shortly."

"Can we move the patient to the dirty cases theatre since you are saying it is now peritonitis?" the theatre nurse asked.

The anesthetist watched quietly at the drama in theatre. This Anesthetist and I had met before. He proceeded to put the patient to sleep as soon as the team was ready. The coverage nurse emerged shortly with a pint of blood and ten litres of saline.

Hastily, I approached the operating table after being gowned in a long green priestly robe. I cleaned the patient's abdomen with three different solutions in a ceremonial manner. The theatre nurse assisted me to cover the patient head to toe. The abdomen could be seen through a window in the abdominal drape we had used.

At 10pm, the operation was finally under way. I cut through the patient's skin from the sternum down to the pubis symphysis. Once inside the abdominal cavity, I was greeted by a sea of pus.

"Do you see why I wanted twelve litres of saline?" I said looking at the coverage nurse who had stayed to witness the operation.

"I see doctor," he answered.

"Do you have to waste so much water when saline is scarce? Couldn't you just suck out the pus using the suction machine? We have serious shortages of fluids in this hospital," the theatre nurse offered an argument.

"My dear nurse, the outcome of this disease is directly proportional to how thorough you washed the abdomen during surgery. I reviewed a patient in the morning, called Rhoda. She is admitted to your Gynecology ward. She has had two operations and she is going to have a third one tomorrow. Do you know why?" I asked looking at the theatre nurse.

"No. Maybe her immune system is weak," she answered.

"She is coming because you washed her abdominal cavity with only one litre of Ringer's Lactate. She was inadequately treated. She now has tertiary peritonitis. It is a miracle she is still alive. Cutting up someone's abdomen is not the treatment for peritonitis. Treatment is washing this abdomen thoroughly and copiously with every drop you got; and where possible, identifying the source of the problem, such as a perforated intestine, perforated appendix or perforated peptic ulcer. I don't know what this guy has. We will search for the usual suspects first," I lectured the poor nurse.

"Ba Sir, what is peritonitis?" a porter they called Yikolo asked. He was keenly observing the operation and wondered what peritonitis was.

(Medical Jargon below [*in italics*], may skip without loss to story flow)

"Mr. Yikolo, *Peritonitis is an inflammatory response to peritoneal injury. Injury results in an influx of protein rich fluid, activation of the complement cascade, up-regulation of peritoneal mesothelial cell activity and invasion of the peritoneum with polymorph nuclear neutrophils and macrophages. There is stimulation of cytokine and chemokine production. Bacteria are opsonised and killed by white blood cells and cleared through the lymphatics. The anatomic origin of bacterial contamination and microbiological findings are no major predictors of outcome. However, the preoperative physiological derangement, the surgical clearance of the infectious focus and the response to treatment are established prognostic factors,"* I answered smiling at Mr. Yikolo.

"Ba sir, say it in Chimambwe or English please," Mr. Yikolo protested.

"Yikolo, Yikolo, you are just a Porter, don't trouble the doctor, he will just confuse you," one of the people in theatre rebuked the Porter.

"Leave Yikolo alone," I intervened. "He is a vital member of this treatment team. Never look down on any member of the care team. No matter how humble their job description may appear, it is vital to complete the care chain. If I asked the Principle Nursing Officer to empty that suction bottle full of pus over there, she would probably feel insulted. Yet this man Yikolo, he would do it with a smile on his face. Teach him, don't brush him aside."

"Thank you doctor for telling them, these people think my job is not important. I also had wanted to become a doctor when I was young," Yikola answered and went, majestically, to empty the suction bottle full of pus.

"My first definition was intended for your doctors. I feel sad none is here to assist in this operation. This was intended to be a platform to exchange and share knowledge and skills. I was sent here for mentorship. I hope it won't turn out to be a vacation for your doctors," I commented looking at the coverage nurse.

"Should I call them?" the coverage asked.

"Leave them, Yikona is here." I answered smiling.

"It is Yikolo doctor," the coverage nurse corrected me.

"Very well then, Yikolo; now, peritonitis is inflammation of the peritoneum. The peritoneum is a silk like membrane that lines our inner abdominal wall and covers the organs within our abdomen. Peritonitis is usually due to a bacterial or fungal infection. It can also result from any rupture or perforation in your abdomen, or as a complication of other medical conditions."

I showed Yikola the peritoneum in the patient's abdomen and quickly turned my attention to search for the likely causes. I inspected the entire length of small intestines looking for perforations caused by typhoid. I then meticulously examined the appendix; however I found it to be normal by my naked eye inspection. I then directed my search to the stomach to look for perforated ulcers. I found none.

"Fuma fuma konsi kunoli; Konsi kuno fiseme nimakuzana *(Come out come out wherever you are…wherever you are hiding, I am coming to get you)*," I announced in Chimambwe beaming with excitement at the complex surgery I was wrestling with.

I then switched my focus to the patient's Liver. The theatre nurse watched anxiously.

"I didn't know you spoke Mambwe doc," she remarked surprised.

"Good Lord, there you are!" I exclaimed when I saw the source of the infection.

"You found it, where is the source of infection?" the Anesthetist asked glad the operation would now enter the end game and come to a close.

"Checkmate; I found the Ghost. I think the gods sent this affliction to test me," I announced looking at the anaesthetist. "This boy has empyema of the gall bladder. The entire porta hepatis is inflamed. It is a jungle down there. A Cholecystectomy is unthinkable in our case. This boy is too ill, he was in septic shock. Yikolo, empyema of the Gallbladder or Suppurative Cholecystitis refers to a rare condition in which the Gallbladder is filled with pus. I have never met it in my fourteen years of practice. I have only read about it. This is my first."

"All that smelly pus I emptied in the suction bottle came from his gallbladder," Yikolo answered shaking his head.

"His Gallbladder is perforated. It has a gangrenous patch at its base," I spelt out complications I had uncovered.

"What are you going to do doc?" Mr. Njhovu the anaesthetist asked visibly concerned about the turn the operation was likely to take. It was now, 11pm and he was tired.

"It would be stupid to try to perform a heroic Cholecystectomy in a patient this ill. I will decompress his gall bladder and perform a cholecystostomy instead. Rapture of the gallbladder has a mortality rate of 30%." I gave my unwavering signature decision. "Yikolo, a cholecystostomy is a procedure where a stoma or mouth or opening is created in the gallbladder, which can facilitate placement of a tube for drainage. It is sometimes used in cases of cholecystitis in which the patient is too ill, and there is a need to delay or defer Cholecystectomy."

Having said this, I asked the nurse to pass me a kidney dish. I then proceeded to decompress the gallbladder. It had grown to the size of an adult's gloved fist. Four hundred milliliters of foul smelling pus came oozing out. I placed a tube inside the gallbladder and secured it. I passed the tube out of the abdomen via another opening on the abdominal wall and attached a collecting bag. Pus could be seen draining immediately. Satisfied with this plumbing I had done, I asked the nurse to prepare the water for washing the interior of the abdomen and all the organs. I washed the patient's abdomen, Liver, spleen, gallbladder, stomach and all the intestines with twelve litres of saline. I was beaming with satisfaction as I did this.

"We are not here to look after fluids; we are here to look after patients. I think hospitals are forgetting their core business nowadays. Every hospital I go to, I find health workers worried about intravenous fluids instead of worrying about their patients. Let us worry about our patients; let he whose job is to supply fluids to the hospitals worry about his job. He is paid for that. Replace him if he is failing in his job. If people should die due to lack of fluids, reflect it in your hospital reports and let the erring officers be punished for negligence of office by public servant. It would be sad to have to write a death certificate; cause of death, No Fluids in the Hospital," I let out a triumphant smirk at my team and scrubbed down.

I concluded the operation notes and sent the patient to the ward.

I left Abercorn Community Hospital (ACH) at midnight and headed for my cozy room at Giza. I was tired. Once at the Inn, I took a long hot shower and reflected on Rhoda, a patient inadequately treated for peritonitis. By the time sleep got to me, it was 2am.

In Search of

I met Mrs. Mwikisa at a local church in Choma town. I was **invited** by her congregation to give a talk on high blood pressure. At the close of the presentation I shared my experiences of what I called 'when God's children pray, strange things happen that medical science cannot explain'. I shared very briefly two stories from this book.

Unknown to me, was a 43yr old woman, listening attentively to my tales. If the congregation did not take me serious, she did.

After the talk, I stood outside greeting and being greeted by the members of this wonderful congregation. As is the case with many doctors, my conversations soon took the form of; 'doctor this, me doctor that....' And waiting patiently for her turn was a lady with a huge deforming Tumor in her left arm pit.

She narrated to me her ten year ordeal at various hospitals seeking for a cure; she had visited every reputable hospital around the country, she had been to Choma General Hospital and seen a good surgeon there. She had been to a mine hospital and attended by a Fellow of the college of surgeons of America.

At UTH, she saw a vascular surgeon. Then she turned her quest to mission hospitals, however here too she was turned back owing to her dangerously high blood pressure.

"All these big hospitals and honorable surgeons, there is something dreadfully anomalous about this tumor," I thought to myself.

"Why wouldn't they operate?" I asked.

"They would turn me back from theatre saying my BP was too high and I couldn't be operated on," she answered with a searching look on her face.

"Was that all?" I probed further unsatisfied with the blood pressure story.

"They also told me the Arm pit had large blood vessels and nerves and operations in this part of the body were precariously complicated," her face dropped as she narrated this. "One of the doctors I saw told me the swelling in my arm pit was a breast."

I thought I saw a tear on the corner of her eye. I couldn't help but ask to examine her arm pit parasitic monster tumor right there. She stretched out her hand to me. I grabbed it at the elbow and ran my fingers up her arm pit. It was the size of a water melon.

"Mm," I murmured. "We can remove it."

She looked at me in disbelief. I knew she thought I was bluffing. I invited her to see me at the hospital for a thorough surgical examination.

Later that evening, I explored all the worst case scenarios I would be faced with if I went ahead and operated on Mrs. Mwikisa. The words of my professor of surgery echoed deafeningly in my ears;

"It takes five years to learn how to operate and twenty years to learn when not to operate."

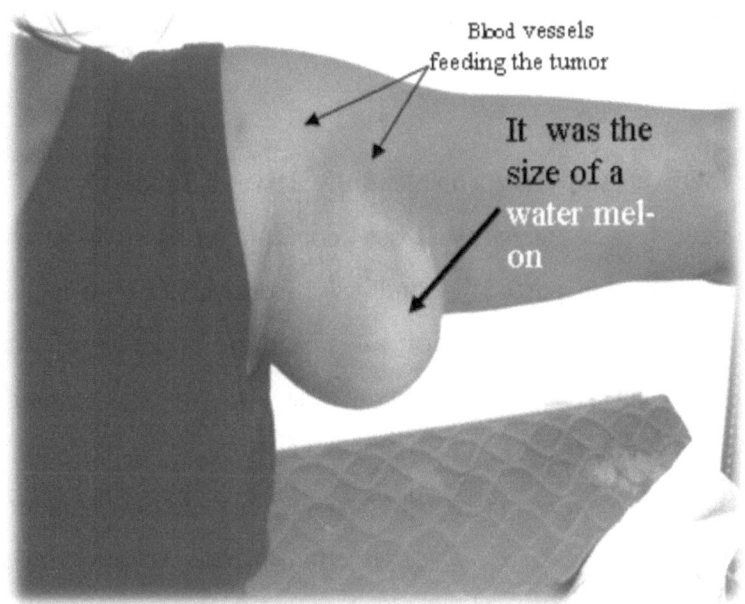

Blood vessels feeding the tumor

It was the size of a water melon

Was this "a leave alone matter" or was this Linda distress call....

In the dead of night, I pondered deeply on the surgery I was daring to take on. I could easily walk away from my impetuous decision to operate. I was committing myself to doing an operation that the learned consultant surgeons had walked away citing high blood pressure as a bad omen.

I practiced surgery under the principle that medicine was not a platform for acts of heroism but a unique vocation akin to an act of worship.

Top on my worst case scenario list was infection. Somehow, I wasn't afraid of her high blood pressure and I wasn't going to allow it to be a deterrent. For another professor of surgery had taught me that the Human body was like an onion; it has layers. With meticulous surgery, you can avoid injury to important structures anywhere in the 'human Onion'. However post surgery infection was a potential hazard and an ideal leave it alone matter.

With this unsavory scenario playing out deep in my mind, I allowed sleep to consume me.

***

The following day passed uneventfully. It was a Sunday.

The new week came and went but I couldn't get Mrs. Mwikisa off my mind. Each day that passed I found myself drawn to revise the detailed Anatomy of the Shoulder and arm pit. I read the pages of my Anatomy text books filled with nostalgia for my days at Medical School in the University of Zambia.

Dissections of the upper limb earned me the nick name Lord Zuckerman from classmates. The dissection manual we used was written by Lord Zuckerman. Thirteen years had passed since.

One bright Sunday afternoon, a month before I met Mrs. Mwikisa, I was called to the hospital to attend to an Emergency. The nurse that made the call told me it was a mining injury needing urgent suturing in theatre because the patient was bleeding and losing lots of blood.

I hurried to the hospital hoping to throw a couple of stitches at the bleeding vessels and be back. I was feeling much like a plumber invited to seal a leak on a horse pipe.

I was horribly wrong….

It turned out to be a major injury requiring extended surgery. The nurse obviously didn't look at the injured man when she made the call. It was beyond belief this man was alive at all.

His right arm had been caught in a rotating machine that almost dismembered him. The bones of his right shoulder had been crushed to fragments. His muscles that move the shoulder scythed. The major blood vessels and nerves that traverse the arm pit had been cut. This pitiless machine entered his shoulder and arm pit like a combination of a welder's torch and a butcher's cutter. Muscles and blood vessels melted in its path. It was unbelievable he had survived a seven hours agonizing journey to the hospital. Under natural circumstances, he would have died from massive torrential bleeding.

Clinically, his hand was dead. It needed an advanced vascular and orthopedic unit to dare stitching it back. However, this was in a third world hospital, attempt to stitch up a potentially dead limb would result in the death of the patient.

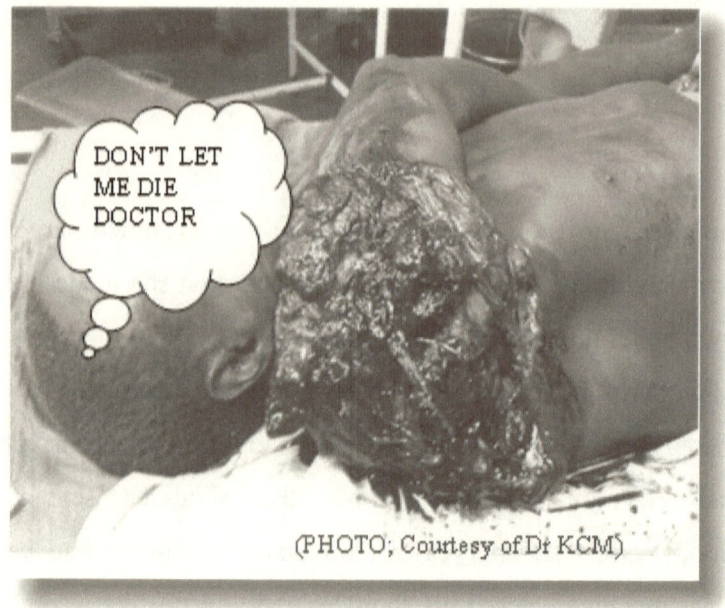

(PHOTO; Courtesy of Dr KCM)

Seeing this I made a diagnosis of traumatic amputation of the right shoulder and speedily made the decision to remove the limb completely from his body. An operation called Amputation. This involved entering deep into the joint itself and cutting off all the grilled dead muscles and ligaments. There was no time for revision.

I hastily phoned a friend, a certified trauma surgeon, 200km away at Livingstone Hospital. I described my predicament. He promptly agreed with the decision to amputate and advised a quick operation to prevent the patient from going into lung shock.

I called the patient's supervisor and relatives to explain this horrible treatment plan.

"I am sorry we can't save his limb," I told them plainly. "It is a miracle he made it to hospital. He is still very critical."

"What are his chances," his supervisor at work asked.

It was a somber scene. His pregnant wife mourned uncontrollably at hearing this news.

He survived the surgery and went on to be discharged out of hospital without infection within two weeks.

Several weeks later after my lecture at the holy church of Choma, I ran into a teacher that knew the woman afflicted by an armpit tumor for ten years. I asked him to remind her about the hospital appointment I had given her. She turned up the following week and was admitted for blood pressure control.

The day of surgery arrived like winter. It was a   mixture of chilling anxiety and exuberant excitement for me. Was this going to be the end of her search for a cure or a mirage on the horizon she had gazed on for the ten years? She handed me her bulky file. It was a wonder to marvel at.

"I have stolen all my files at the hospitals I have been to," she laughed as she walked into theatre. She looked very calm as she was led to our operating table.

I was young and looked like her son. The previous surgeons were much older than her. They were distinguished Surgeons in their respective specialties. I was a Bachelor's degree in Surgery; however she looked calm in my theatre. A monitor was hooked to her arm and at a place of a button, it sprung to life. After a few beeps and chimes, the monitor displayed a normal blood pressure across its screen.

"It seems your blood pressure won't be complaining today," I smiled.

"You made me feel at home," she giggled.

I picked my razor sharp scalpel and descended onto to the tumor with the surreptitiousness of a stealth hunter. I worked at the mass assisted by a meticulous theatre nurse named Dorothy. The corner of my eye kept vigil of the blood pressure monitor. It remained normal. The nurse handed me tissue scissors, artery forceps and in just a few minutes, surgery was over.

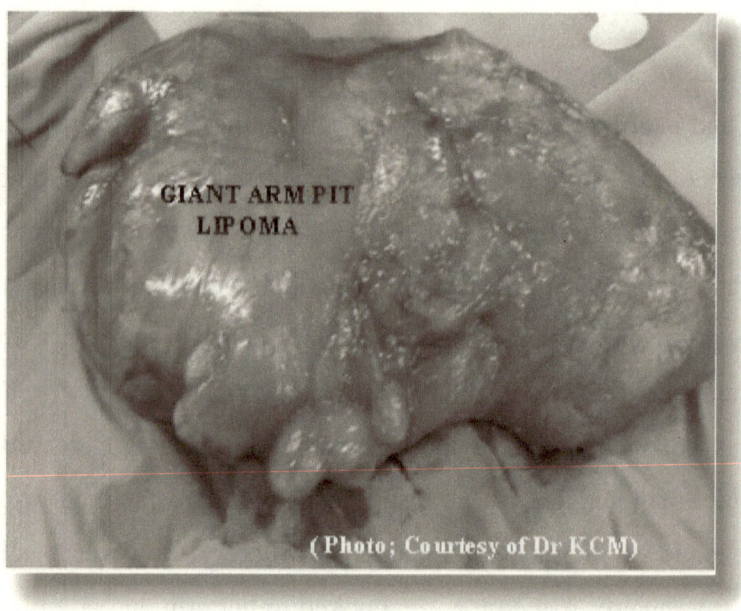

GIANT ARM PIT LIPOMA

(Photo; Courtesy of Dr KCM)

The massive tumor, about a kilo in weight popped out and exited her arm pit like a gigantic alien maggot.

It Left behind a large cavity that I easily closed.

Her ten year search had finally come to an END.

EFCON

After a light lunch in the hospital cafeteria, I hurried to the Gynecology ward to see Rhoda. She had not received blood and her condition was now desperate. The student doctors; Jessy, Joan and Serena had joined me for lunch.

They followed me to learn how to manage severe anemia in a rural community hospital. We were met by Dr Kalunda in the wide corridor leading to the children's ward.

"You girls don't want to see me nowadays," he teased the medical students and stopped to greet Me.

"How can we come to see you when you don't buy us lunch," Serena answered giggling.

"We just had a wonderful Lunch with our new teacher," said Joan laughing.

"I can see you are fascinated working with your wonderful teacher," Dr Kalunda remarked. "He taught me too you know."

"I think they are excellent students," I said.

"I think you are a good teacher," Kalunda answered smiling.

Just then, an Ambulance from the district office veered in. We all turned to see what it had brought. A nurse and another person emerged shortly aiding a patient who could hardly stand. My quick mind noticed the patient could not support her own head. She was dragging her feet between the shoulders rushing her to Maternity.

"Doc, that patient is in shock," I said rushing to check on the patient. "Put her down. Lay her on the floor."

The nurse and her assistance put the patient down wondering what was going on.

"We are rushing her to Maternity," the nurse answered after placing the patient down.

"No, you are rushing her to her death," I snapped at the poor nurse.

Meanwhile Dr Kalunda was kneeling by the body on the floor checking for pulses. She had no running Intravenous Access.

"Which health post are you from?" I asked.

"The patient is suffering from anemia in pregnancy. She came to our centre last night. She was just ok," the poor nurse answered.

"I think she is just hungry," the nurse's assistance answered.

"And who are you?" I asked the male assistant. He was in his late 30s.

"I am the community health assistance," he answered proudly looking at me.

"You were right doc, this woman is in shock. All her peripheries are cold and clammy. Unfortunately, we don't have blood in the hospital," Dr Kalunda explained with audible quiver in his voice.

I knelt down and examined the patient. I rose immediately, "This woman has a ruptured uterus. Dr Joan, rush bring two gray Cannulars from the ward, Dr Jessica bring surgical gloves and two litters saline, Serena bring a stretcher." I gave clear military orders to my assiduous young doctors.

By now, this make shift Corridor Emergency Room had attracted several other student doctors; Agnes, Sipho, Natasha, Esther and Kaluba gathered eager to lend a hand.

"Doctors, we are at DEFCON 2," I explained the situation to the new arrivals.

"Defcon; is she dead?" Esther asked wondering what I meant by DEFCON 2.

"Defense Readiness Condition, DEFCON, is an alert state used by the United States Military. We could call ours ERCON; for Emergency Readiness Condition but I like the sound of DEFCON," I explained. "Unfortunately this case is an Emergency Failed Condition, EFCON."

Johnny Mbala arrived pushing a trolley with Serena. Sr Agnes Francis was a beautiful student Nun, always calm and collected. She arrived carrying specimen bottles to collect samples for the laboratory. O'Neil appeared at the corridor emergency room holding a urine bag.

I sent Kaluba and Felix Katongo to inform theatre staff to prepare to receive a very sick woman and to set the theatre alertness to DEFCON 2.

"Shouldn't we first take her to Maternity?" Johnny Mbala asked.

"My dear Dr Johnny this is war. We are at DEFCON 2; we are going straight to theatre from here. We can't afford to waste another hour, we could lose this patient." I answered. "Sr Francis, go to the blood bank. Tell them Dr Ordinary Zambian wants five collecting bags for blood *IMMEDIATELY.*"

Now, Johnny had a long bearded chin that gave him an exceptionally pious look. He was an unusually quiet fellow with a keen eye. He had wanted to become a priest but the desires of his flesh prevented him. He found he was not cut out for a long lonely life of celibacy. There was rumour among his fellow students that he had run away from a Tibetan Monastery. He loved Sr Francis a great deal and often teased her. She invoked memories in him that conspired against the prospective Father Johnny, and probably a future pope.

"Are you planning on conducting auto transfusion?" Dr Kalunda asked. "I am coming to see. I have never seen this being done."

"Most certainly; there are four litters of free blood inside her belly. I am not planning on wasting it," I answered beaming with excitement.

Joan's saline bottles were, by now, running down the patient's veins. Torrents of rain had not let off since morning. The exotic trees that adorned the façade of Abercorn Community Hospital swayed beautifully in the Rain. Collection of drizzles from the roof ran down the drainage on the edge of the corridor like an agitated shallow seasonal stream. A haze could be seen over the surrounding areas. Old Location, Kampompo and new Location Townships were covered in thick fog. It was freezing outside. This was the weather that had attracted the white settlers to Abercorn. With average annual temperature of 18.7 degrees, Mbala was truly a seat of London weather.

***

My team and I arrived in theatre shortly. We placed our patient on supplemental oxygen and continued to stabilize her for surgery. The theatre nurse was busy arranging her instruments on the operating table.

- Meantime, I ran through the steps for auto transfusion. I warned my students what they were about to witness was not standard practice. I told them, in rural Zambia; desperate situations called for desperate solutions at the front line of emergency rural health care delivery.

"Emergency health care in the rural is not different from care during armed conflict or war," I explained. "The blood we are about to use has many impurities. It is mixed with amniotic fluid, Vernix Caseosa and possibly meconium. She may even have Vernix Caseosa Peritonitis, a rare but serious complication seen following Caesarean section."

"What is Vernix Caseosa?" Joan asked.

"Is the waxy or cheese-like white substance found coating the skin of newborn human babies," I answered.

"How does Vernix Caseosa peritonitis start," Johnny Mbala asked.

"It is thought to occur as a result of spillage of amniotic fluid and or meconium into the maternal peritoneal cavity. Uterine rapture in our patient has done exactly that." I answered.

"Here are the blood collecting bags. They gave me eight giving sets,"

"Well done sister," I complimented Sr. Francis. "Joan and Jessica I will need you to stand next to me on my right but mind the sterile field. You will hold the filtering chamber for the blood. It will run down a giving set attached to it into a receiving bag. Felix and Kaluba will be holding the receiving bag or reinfusion bag. They will pass the collected pints of blood to Agnes and Johnny who will connect the bag to the line running into the patient's veins and pump the blood back into the patient's vascular compartment. Musonda, you will squeeze the pint of blood on the right and Kaoma, will squeeze the one on the left. Dr Kalunda, you will scrub in with me. You can wash and prep the patient's abdomen while I check whether these guys have got their roles well."

The anaesthetist was impressed with my sense of calm leadership in the face of an emergency. It gave the team confidence even when it was clear this was a dire situation.

"Doc, won't that lead to Vernix Caseosa SIRS?" Agnes asked.

"Systemic Inflammatory Response Syndrome, that is right Sr Francis," I answered.

"It is like Jumping out of the frying pan into the Fire," Father Johnny Mbala remarked. Every one burst out laughing.

"Jonny, do you know what your name means?" I asked.

"No sir," he answered.

"It means one who has no fear; having courage; having a fine appearance. Gallant, courteous, like an ideal knight; someone with a special charm or allure that inspires allegiance or devotion; One of the, if not the coolest person someone will encounter in their life time. The most interesting man in the room at all times," I explained and everyone burst out laughing.

"OMG...no wonder I hear people say; *He's hung like Johnny!*" Joan remarked.

"I think the beard makes him the most interesting student in this theatre," Sr Francis teased him. "He looks like he jumped out of a frying pan himself."

"I am the coolest person you will ever encounter in your life time," he answered with a grin. "Doc, with no proper blood in the hospital this is definitely a frying pan-fire jumping desperado."

(Medical Jargon below [*in italics*], may skip without loss to story flow)

"You could call it that; only, in our situation, my dear Father Dr Johnny, the fire isn't burning yet. We may have a window of escape before the blaze engulfs the pan. In the case of Vernix Caseosa Peritonitis, it presents as an acute abdomen days to weeks after a seemingly uncomplicated caesarean section. Only a few cases have been reported to date. *The pathophysiology of* Vernix Caseosa Peritonitis *is incompletely understood. Histological examinations of biopsy specimens reveal anucleate squamous cells along with lanugo hair and foreign body giant cell reaction. The diagnosis must be considered in cases of post CS acute abdomen. Your question Sr Francis, this may be the first case of Vernix Caseosa Systemic Inflammatory Response Syndrome, VC-SIRS. It has never been reported in the literature. We are familiar with Amniotic Fluid embolism, a lethal killer.* We can only pray, our patient survives the fire," I explained stepping onto the operating table.

"Father Johnny will pray for her. She will just be alright," Sr Agnes remarked smirking at Johnny.

The nurse passed me the surgical knife. I made a short vertical incision below the patient's umbilicus. I dissected my way into the abdominal cavity carefully. There was no drop of blood to be found in the tissues of the abdomen. The patient was completely white. She had bled massively internally. A midwife 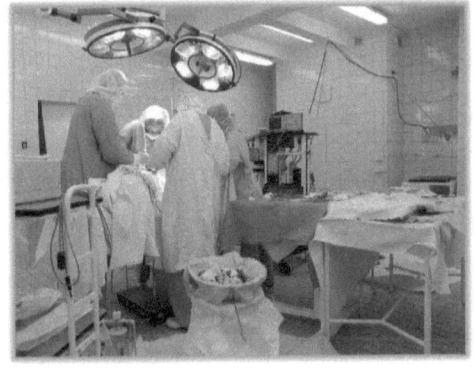 had joined the team. She walked leisurely into theatre knowing the baby was dead.

"Doctor, there is no blood in the blood bank. They said the patient's hemoglobin was 7g/dl," she reported.

I did not answer her. By now, I had entered the peritoneal cavity. I asked the theatre nurse to pass me a Gallipot. The midwife rushed to turn on the suction machine upon seeing the sea of blood in the patient's abdomen.

"Switch off that machine," the anaesthetist ordered her.

"Dr Jessica and Dr Joan, are we ready?

"We are ready sir,"

I dipped the Gallipot inside the patient's abdomen and filled it with blood. I then poured it into the filter Jessica and Joan were holding. The deep dark red blood ran down plastic tubing into the collecting bag Felix and Kaluba were holding. Soon one unit was ready for use. The priest connected it religiously and ran it down into the patient's veins.

"This looks like an Agricultural irrigation system, a Hydro-Engineering Science Model," Johnny observed.

"That's very true; the incision wound on the abdomen is like a well. The blood represents water. The Galipot is like a bucket for drawing water. And what Joan and Jessica are holding is like a reservoir tank," Serena drew an analogy.

"This is an unconventional system you are observing. The actual system is elaborate; it has a collecting reservoir, like the one Joan is holding, which is connected to a vacuum. To the line of the shed blood is attached a bag containing an anticoagulant. The blood runs down a valve system and is mixed with a wash solution before entering the reinfusion bag such as the one Kaluba and Felix are holding," I explained to my fascinated team.

The midwife was utterly awestruck. She stood at the foot end of the operating table and watched in total bewilderment. By now, the team had collected five pints of blood.

Satisfied with the success of my ingenuity, I turned my attention to the dead baby in the womb. I grabbed it by the legs and passed it to the midwife still attached to the placenta at the umbilicus. It was covered with Vernix Caseosa.

"The waxy or cheese-like white substance coating the skin of the baby is Vernix Caseosa," I explained holding the dead baby in my hands. "Joan, you can go and take a look."

I then turned my attentention to the uterus. It had suffered a wide posterior tear and could not be saved. There was no active bleeding from its edges. The tear extended from an old Caesar wound in front to the back and downwards to the vagina.

***

While I worked frantically to remove the uterus, via an operation called total hysterectomy, the students chatted with the midwife in the neonatal resuscitation unit in the opposite room.

"The baby looks big, was it Mature?" Jessica asked.

"It is 3.5kg," the midwife answered after weighing it. "It was a girl."

"Where is she from? Why couldn't she go to the hospital early? She was a previous Caesar right," Joan asked looking sad.

"She was from Mpulungu," said Johnny

"An Island on lake Tanganyika," Serena answered.

"Poor woman, maternal health services are very poor in that area," Felix remarked.

"Am sure she thought she could deliver at home," said Kaoma.

"She was afraid to go to hospital because of the previous caesarean she had. Many women don't go to hospital even when we advise them to," the midwife told the students.

"Why is it so?" Sipho asked. "Maybe you frighten them."

"They are usually afraid at the prospects of having another operation. I wouldn't be surprised to hear that this woman took traditional labour enhancing drugs," Johnny explained.

"Kaselelele, a traditional Oxytocin, is most likely," the mid wife remarked. "Who is that new doctor you are with? I have never seen him. She must thank God for sending him here. This woman would have died."

"That's Dr Mukonka," Joan answered rolling her eyes. "He is my hero."

While the students chatted with the midwife, I had finished the operation. I washed the patient's abdomen copiously with saline to prevent Vernix Caseosa Peritonitis. I left two drains and proceeded to close the abdomen.

I left the operating room and strode along the wide corridor bemoaning the lack of state of the art Emergency Rooms, ERs and a professional Ambulance Service country wide.

I was tired; it had been a long operation. I stood for a while and stared out through the window on the eastern end of the operating theatre. The lawn outside between the gynecology and surgical wards looked beautiful in the rain. I had forgotten that there was still a drizzle outside.

Stalking the Paranormal

"Rise and Shine, Rise and Shine; it is 0530, time for the morning drill," the announcer's voice echoed from the speakers on the wall.

"Oh no, these people, it is freezing outside. Can't we just skip this morning exercise? This place is cold. I don't remember August ever being this cold. I need to consult an atlas, this could be the Arctic. Where did I put my diary? I haven't written anything down since I arrived."

A surge of high voltage thoughts raced through my mind as I tried to flee the comfy of my bed. I reached for my diary and begun to write;

"It is Wednesday, in the year Nineteen Hundred and Ninety. I am in Kitwe at Mpelembe Secondary School. I arrived three days ago by train in the company of four school mates; Bruce, James, Teddy and Swithurn.

James, Bruce and I are in grade eleven. Teddy is in grade ten. Swithurn aged ten, is the youngest of the group and is in grade eight but has a brain of a senior pupil.

We travelled to attend the national scripture union conference being held at this prestigious school. I am excited to be here. There is one little problem though; we are the only group not accompanied by a Teacher.

One of the conditions to be here was; pupils had to be accompanied by a teacher. We have a very young delegate in our group and we definitely could have used some senior eyes to shepherd us.

None of the teachers were willing to come with us. Actually we don't even have a patron or matron to supervise our activities back at school. The five of us are the committee of the vibrant Kafue Boys Scripture Union. We decided to make the journey hoping the organizers would understand our special case.

This trip is a fruition of three months prayer. The whole of second term we have been praying to be here. We did not have any money to make the trip but God answered our prayer beyond our wildest dreams.

One evening, on a Sunday, we were in prayer during our scheduled scripture union meetings when a Ghanaian teacher walked in. I don't remember him ever having attended our meetings before. We all wondered why he was there. He told us he had something to share with us. So we gave him the platform and were all ears.

"God has sent me to give you this money," he said. He handed us an envelope and left as mysterious as he had appeared. We were ecstatic.

The money was enough to send an entire class for the conference; however the invitation was for five pupils only. This presented us with a new problem. Everyone wanted to attend the conference in Kitwe. We decided God was going to make the selection.

After weeks of prayer, it came to this number…This is how I found myself here with my four friends. We must be one of the richest groups attending this conference.

It is so cold outside that I can't feel my own ears. My fingers and Feet are frozen. I won't be able to go jogging. I think there is ice outside. This is not the Kitwe I was hoping to find. But wait, what is this strange feeling I am getting. I definitely feel as if there is someone I ought to find.

It is becoming clear; I ought to find a pupil in distress. This is confusing. I'll ask the boys; maybe one of them can explain what I am experiencing.

What if this is a message from God? That can't be, why would he want to use a person like me when he has all these pastors and reverends to send. He wouldn't definitely ask a school boy and certainly not me. However, out of curiosity, let me keep this to myself and find this mysterious person.

Where do I even start from, there are over two hundred participants at this conference. Doesn't the bible say that when he sends you, he will also equip you for his work?"

Torrents of nostalgic memories pour through my mind as I begin to write down these events. I have reflected on this experience a million times since.

The call to find this mysterious person was so intriguing that I couldn't decline the challenge, largely because it was simple. I didn't need to build Noah's Ark or go to rebuke an evil king over his immoral ways. I wasn't being asked to march into Nazi Germany to tell Hitler to let the 'Jews go' claiming I have seen a 'talking forest fire'.

I was simply required to walk around within my usual conference program and allow the Spirit to lead. I was not even required to know the full details of this assignment.

This couldn't have been any simpler and probably explains why he picked a school boy to carry it.

I like to think of my practice as a reminiscence of the events that begun on this cold Wednesday morning at Mpelembe Secondary school. Two decades have passed since but for me, it feels to have been just yesterday.

While experiencing this supernatural dimension, I was fulfilling an academic pilgrimage being at Mpelembe that August. Back at school, I was in a pure sciences class and we called ourselves 'Mpelembe boys based at Kafue secondary school. Our Chemistry teacher taught 'A' level chemistry at Mpelembe before coming to Kafue boys secondary. He was so pleased to find such an enthusiastic class deep in the hills of Kafue town. It was he that equated us to his previous 'A' level class at Mpelembe. Pampered like this, we worked even harder not wanting to disappoint our teacher. Three years earlier, I arrived at Kafue having transferred from Kamwala secondary school in Lusaka, for my grade eight.

While in primary school, I had asked God to send me to a school where I would work for him. In the 7th Grade of primary school, I accepted Jesus as my savior and devoted myself to studying the Holy Bible. I must have read it cover to cover a million times. I was fortunate to have been nurtured in an interdenominational fellowship of mature believers.

Kafue Boys Secondary School was notorious for violent acts of mockery on the grade eights. Grade eight was the worst year any pupil spent at this school. It was here, for the first time in my life, I was tortured for being a Christian. On several occasions, evil senior boys asked us to deny Jesus or be tortured for our faith. I could never deny Jesus.

This torture involved anything from being made to roll in muddy pools of water, physical assault, food taken away from you, being made to wash cloths for evil senior pupils every weekend, etc. A grade eight pupil was considered a washing machine by senior pupils.

Many times, we were woken up in the early hours of the morning to go jogging in a full military recruit *like* drill. We were made to carry heavy loads while running and would be made to roll in mud when we failed to complete the set tasks. Sometimes, we were forced to climb a steep incline of a notorious mountain known as Koka Hill.

Three years earlier a pupil died on this same slop. Often our evil captors would be masked and armed to the teeth with an assortment of sticks and whips. They were often eager to use these weapons of iniquity to thwart any mutiny.

I survived the year however I do not recall ever attending the scripture union during my grade eight. I was invited to attend once but was horribly disappointed to find decadent boys who were torturing the grade eights in my dormitory just the previous night, standing sanctimoniously at the pulpit, preaching. I felt betrayed and vowed to distance myself from this reek of hypocrisy.

This was my background when we arrived at Mpelembe. As I recall, I think we each were given a group to lead at the conference. The participants were divided into nineteen groups. I was group leader for Damascus.

Each group competed for points of excellence every day and it was the responsibility of the group leader to see to it that his group earned every available point. Points were awarded for punctuality in all set activities of the day. You lost points by reporting late to venues of set out activities. A minus two demerit was charged on any of your group members late for an activity.

I had figured out the weakest point for all groups was the rise and shine rush hour to the football pitch. Everyone in Damascus knew our secret winning strategy and so I was not going to let down my group that freezing morning.

I got out of bed at 05:42, packed my diary and sprinted for the fields. It was so cold that only a hand full of groups turned up.

As for Damascus, we scored our trade mark straight 22 points. We were fortunate to have only one girl in the group. She turned out to be my course mate in medical school five years later.

I completed our morning fitness drill without a sight of the mystery delegate. The drill was followed by 30min grooming which was never enough for the girls. This always cost us negative two demerits. It was devastating for groups with lots of girls.

I got to the dining hall ahead of everyone that morning. I was not at all hungry; I just wanted to have a very good view of everyone coming in. I thought this would help me pick out my mystery person. Unfortunately, I was not even sure what I was supposed to be looking out for.

Soon, it was time for the morning service and bible study which were followed by a break into various workshops. This day, I decided to attend a workshop on writing from God's word. I had noticed an inclination to writing among my hobbies. The workshop turned out to be extremely fascinating however the stranger chose not to attend this workshop.

At lunch time, I hurried to the dining hall and took a thorough assessment of the participants' hungry faces as they walked in.

"I probably need a gigantic microscopy or a quantum mechanics equation to solve this mystery," I thought to myself as lunch came to a close.

As Noon slipped into evening I grew into despair. I had done well not to have told anyone about this. They would have questioned the god I was listening to. There are too many lying spirits out there.

I was lucky to know the warning about testing all spirits to see whether they were from God.

When you get a conviction to sell your car, your house, your farmland and feel that strong inner urge to donate the money to your local church, make sure you listen carefully before you act. Don't even tell anyone about the conviction you are having. God is not vague in dealing with his children. Wait upon him patiently; he will confirm it to you if it comes from him. Always remember the boundary between Faith and Foolishness can be as thin as a thread of your hair. The bible cautions us to Test the spirits to see whether they are from God.

And so it was, day slipped into dusk however the ghost remained elusive. I was now convinced I had responded to a false alarm. I wasn't at all disappointed with myself. I knew if this was God, he would do it in his own time. My search time was over. I decided to give it one last try. I decided I would enter the dining hall after everyone had gone in that evening. So as the crowds coming for supper thinned out, I decided it was over. I needed to get something to eat. It had been a long cold day.

I joined the queue for the evening meal feeling disappointed. The usher at the door handed me a disc indicating my position on the queue and I rolled it in my hands uninterested in my surroundings. Suddenly my attention was drawn to the number a little girl in front of me was holding. She was about twelve years old and she was holding number eighty two. I was a teenager myself however I felt much older than her.

"Do you know that's the number I had over lunch," I tried to make conversations with the little girl. "You are standing exactly at the position I stood for lunch. What grade are you?"

"I am supposed to have been in grade nine, unfortunately I was sick the whole of last year,' she replied.

"I am sorry to hear that. Did it happen to you when you were a believer in Jesus Christ or before?' I asked.

However she did not answer me. I assumed she hadn't got the question, so I rephrased it and asked again.

"Were you a Christian when you fell ill that long?' She still didn't answer.

It then dawned on me that this could be the person I was searching for. She looked a perfectly normal girl however what I was about to find out terrified me to my bone and changed my life forever.

When we had collected our food, I asked her to sit with me to the restricted section of the dining hall. Boy -Girl eating arrangements were discouraged at this conference. Moreover the section of the dining hall I was proposing we sit was reserved for the form six students at Mpelembe. She obliged and we soon found a table and sat facing each other.

Once we were seated, I again asked my earlier question. I was not sure why she didn't want to answer my questions. She still didn't answer.

I sat on the wooden chair and waited for her to say something. I nibbled on my piece of chicken while watching and waiting. She scarcely touched her food during this impending stalemate.

We sat till people started leaving the dining hall. No one came to enquire why we sat on this prohibited section of the dining hall. They simply watched and I paid no attention.

Finally, she sat up and stared me straight in the face with the coldest look I have ever seen. There was no trace of emotion in that face. My mind failed to capture a mental image of her real face. It was as if I was gazing at the face of death itself.

Goose pimples sprung up my arms and I begun to freeze as I had at dawn of that day. She kept her face focused on me like an evil spirit sent from the underworld. I then became aware of an evil chilling presence that had come to take over her life. I sat face to face with Lucifer himself. He had taken over her body and he was trying to devour mine too. A spiritual battle was on.

Fortunately, the one in me was greater than the one possessing her. I wished I had spiritual eyes to actually watch this spiritual battle for souls raging around our tiny dining table.

She lost all control of her body, taken over like this, to the dictates of forces of the underworld. The feeling she was having is quite similar to a familiar feeling you get sometimes when you have had a nightmare and are trying to awake. You try to shout for help but no voice comes out. You try to move your legs and arms but you can't. It is the most frightening experience to have. You get trapped inside your own body.

After what appeared to have been millennia, she finally spoke up;

"I am demon possessed, can you help me? This is the reason I came for this conference. I want to be delivered from this torment I am in. Please help me."

My heart missed a beat and I swallowed hard. I didn't know what to do. I thought of running away. I could sense the air around me was tense. My hair stood on end. A legion of demons was holding the poor girl hostage.

She narrated how during preaching her heart pounded hard and how she would become breathless. When this happened, she would hurriedly run outside and stay far from the reach of the prayers and the praise and worship.

She told me things a girl of 12 shouldn't know.

While I was pondering how I was going to deal with this legion of demons, a pastor passed by to where we sat. I rose up immediately and narrated my sticky situation. He asked me to arrange a rendezvous with the little girl and hand her to them after the evening service. I returned to the table and reassured her I would help her get deliverance.

"By the way, my name is Kelly J Song. You can simply call me Kelly. I am not quite sure I even introduced myself. Forgive me for harassing you with those questions before we were even introduced."

"That's ok, I didn't feel harassed. I saw that you wanted to help me. I actually felt very safe the moment you started talking with me. It felt as if I was surrounded by a strong wall of protection. My name is Linda. None of my friends in the group know I suffer from demon possession. You are the first human I have been able to talk to about my problem. Each time I tried to talk to other people, my mouth would be locked and I would fail to say anything."

We left the dining hall and arranged to meet at 10pm at the entrance to the conference hall. She hurried to find her friends and I headed for my room to pray and prepare for battle at 22hrs. I didn't care anymore about earning a demerit for being late for the evening service, so I walked slowly humbled by what God had revealed to me. I didn't know then that this supernatural call to find someone in distress would characterize my practice of medicine many years later.

I walked to my room pondering the complex subject of Demons and

Satanism. I recalled how pupils at Kafue boys, and in many other schools, would run away from the dormitory alleging there was a demon in the room or that there was a Satanist in school and they couldn't sleep. We would go to pray in these rooms and invite the affected pupils to join the scripture union to learn the power of God for their lives.

Today, the fear of the so called Satanists in our schools and homes has reached alarming levels. Learning, in most high schools, has from time to time been disrupted by pupils suspecting their teachers of being Satanists.

You hardly ever hear of such narrow minded medieval thinking in higher institutions of learning such as schools of Engineering, Law, Business and Medicine. It would appear that the superstitions surrounding Satanism reflect people's level of Civilization, Educational background and ignorance of the power of the spirit of God for their lives.

After prayer, I headed for the Rendezvous with Linda.

We met as planned and she was immediately taken away in the company of senior Pastors and Reverends.

I met Linda the following morning looking totally reborn. She saw me at a distance and came running towards me.

"I am free now. I have been set free and I have accepted Jesus Christ as my personal savior. Thank you for coming to find me," she said with tears rolling down her cheeks.

She wiped her eyes and a wide smile lit up her face. This was the last I saw of Linda and would probably never meet again.

The Physical Linda I met in Kitwe was afflicted by spiritual illness.

The Spiritual Linda I meet in my practice of Medicine is afflicted with Physical illness.

I have lived by this paradoxical paradigm ever since.

Sword of Damocles

The year is 2004. She walked into my consultation room with the tranquility of Mona Lisa, the 16th century bravura oil painting by Leonardo Da Vinci. She was calm however to the trained eye she was visibly riding a tempestuous tide.

There were several people that day in the outpatient department. An ox-cart, drawn by two large brown oxen, stood in the ambulance parking lot. It brought a critically ill antenatal mother. Several bicycles were parked outside. The villagers wore dirty old work cloths. I wondered what such a pretty young lady was doing in my village gynecology clinic.

"Welcome to Macha Mission Hospital. I am Dr Siyajanika Hambilwi Abana. How might I help you?" I ventured a conversation.

"Thank you Sir; I am sorry I can't say your name correctly, it is very long," she answered handing me a referral letter addressed to the Specialist at my hospital.

"You may call me Dr SHA," I smiled.

"SHA…" she repeated perplexed.

"It means keep out of reach of children," I smiled shifting my attention to her letter.

Mission hospitals across the country were reputed to be offering the highest standard of health care in the country. Many patients travelled from all over the country in search of this care.

I handed her back the letter and begun to explain.

"I see you have come a long way Mercy, do you have relatives in this area?"

She had been referred from a clinic in Chirundu to see a gynecologist for a disease they called primary amenorrhea. She was 23 and going on 24 in a few months. She had never had a menstrual period. All her three young sisters aged 21, 19 and 16 had their first menses by ages of 11, 13 and 14 respectively.

Now turning 24, this was beginning to worry her.

She was betrothed, in college, to a handsome young man and in nine months time they were planning to wed. He was six years older than her and eager to settle down and raise a family. He worked as a tourism logistic manager for an international tourism company based in Livingstone. He had graduated two years earlier with a degree in Business Administration and Marketing.

Without her menses, she was not sure she would be a mom. She taught Mathematics at a local high school but carried herself like an Arts and culture teacher. While most Science teachers paid little attention to their dressing, this mademoiselle gave dress the detail of a model. She wore a modest purple dress cut from expensive linen yet blended inconspicuously in this conservative rural community.

The dress's overlapping V shaped neck reinforced with delicately cut out white semi lunar flaps just concealed her virgin breasts in a laced white brassiere. The top was further reinforced with an independent piece of garment that spread from the back of her neck, down her shoulders to cover her long beautiful arms beyond her elbows. This garment could be drawn right in front of her chest to conceal it completely. It could also be drawn upwards to cover her head leaving only her face or any part she trusted you to behold.

This piece transformed her into a modest religious beauty in an instance. When dropped, it rested on her waist held by her elbows and exposed her sleeveless bare back tunic. Drawn this way, gave her a seductive look rivaled only by Cleopatra, Queen and last Pharaoh of Egypt.

"Queen Sheba of Ethiopia must have worn one of these when she seduced the wise King Solomon," I thought to myself and added, almost audibly and caring less on the accuracy of my history facts. "Cleopatra too must have used this tactic to seduce the might Julius Caesar in 48 BC. Caesar was an extremely Adulterous Psychopath." Legend has it that she seduced him wrapped in a carpet.

Clothed in one of these impersonation gowns, a lady presents a saintly air of vulnerability, defenselessness and innocence to her prey at first contact and in a matter of seconds draws it away as she wins their trust to reveal an irresistible devilish inner being wrapped in an evening garb.

Being a young Doctor myself and a novice on many matters of women psych, I had been warned to beware of young girls and ladies that malingered in gynecology clinics in search of a doctor lover.

Some, truly obsessed by this prospect, would fake any horrendous gynecological disease just to book an audience with an unsuspecting male Doctor in the examination room.

Mercy was an upright girl. Her story would profoundly affect my practice and change her life forever. I explained to her that the Hospital did not have a specialist Doctor she had been sent to see. There was a visiting doctor, a Canadian gynecologist that once visited Macha. It was probably this doctor, those that referred her had heard about. I told her I was at this hospital for rural posting and that I had only recently graduated from medical school.

"I can see you if you don't mind a non specialist doctor with a fun name," I offered.

Her disappointment was palpable in the room. You could see the discontent on her face as she held on to her independent piece of garment like an Arab woman engulfed by desert winds. After a prolonged moment of indecision, she agreed to be seen by me. I guessed she figured there would be nothing to be lost; she had already made the journey.

Seeing the reluctance and apprehension on her face, I decided to skip the physical examination and sent her for a pelvic scan instead.

I returned from lunch that day not expecting to find Mercy. Quite on the contrary, I found an excited patient waiting eagerly for me. I wondered what had gotten into her.

"You look very happy Mercy! Did you have a lovely lunch?" I asked curious to know what was making her so happy.

"I met pastor E in radiology department and he told me all about you. He was confident you would help me. I am excited I travelled this far to see you," she replied with her eyes glowing with excitement.

Pastor E and his wife were radiographers and performed all ultra sound scans at the hospital. This young couple was a blessing to work with. They spent time with their patients and were always on hand to help those in need.

"Ah! You met pastor E. He is always too kind, isn't he? But he always exaggerates about me to my patients," I laughed. "We are merely vessels in God's hands honey. We can only do what is human; Divinity is to be left for God."

"I agree with Pastor E, you are a very humble man Dr SHA," she smiled.

We walked along the concrete walkway from the radiology department. We passed the operating room to our left. Several patients and their relatives sat under mango trees in front of the male ward. The HIV pandemic was at its peak. Frail humans, reduced to skin and bone, lay on mats everywhere. For many this day, would be the last sunshine they would see. They were too feeble to face the demons that would be lurking in the shadows when the sun went down. The price of antiretroviral drugs was still out of reach for the locals. Mercy appeared to understand the desperation on the faces of many patients we passed on the way to my office.

"Could I see the ultra sound report?' I asked once we got to the office.

"Sure," she said. "I nearly forgot about the scan. I feel fine already just talking to you. What's wrong with all those ill patients we passed along the way? Are they AIDS patients?"

"It is AIDS, you are right," I agreed. "Unfortunately there are no drugs yet. Patients have to buy their own medicines. I only hope treatment will be free soonest or entire families will be wiped out."

I turned my attention to the ultrasound report. Pastor E was a detailed and thorough sonographer. His reports were written in clear legible Lucida handwriting and always made interesting reading.

The detail on this particular report however, was like a Jury's unsavory verdict. It stated that Mercy's Uterus and tubes were ABSENT. He went on to elaborately report presence of two ovoid structures in her abdomen and gave precise measurements. This prompted me to suggest a thorough physical Examination and I carefully explained what this involved. To which she obliged.

I moved her to a warm gynecology examination room and asked the nurse to help her take off all her cloths. I then asked her to walk about in the room while I looked for telltale signs for her strange affliction.

She didn't appear at all embarrassed by this; instead she roamed about the room in full control of her figure with an elegant model like persona. I then asked the nurse to assist her lie on the examination couch.

Nothing was remarkable until I got to the Pelvic Examination. The external genitalia; labia, clitoris, urethral opening and general shape were normal but the vagina.

The birth canal was absent. This was a frightening finding, one I wasn't prepared to disclose to her or anyone else at that point.

She explained how, at one clinic, a doctor she had consulted told her that he could cut open her birth canal with a scalpel and was told she would be a woman like everyone else. I warned her never to return to this mad man. He obviously didn't know the difference between an imperforate hymen and Mercy's condition.

She also narrated the ordeal she had been through from her family to consult traditional healers. They believed that an evil spirit had cast a spell on her and closed her womanhood. She was told a portion of traditional medicine could break this spell.

She revealed to me an incidence where a terrifying witchdoctor had wanted to use a sharp pointed magic spear, heated red Hot, to literally burrow a vagina into her perineum. She was so terrified by this treatment that she vowed never to see a witchdoctor in her life ever again.

We concluded our discussion and bade farewell. In a month's time, I was leaving Macha for the University of Zambia, School of Medicine. I had been offered a place to study a Masters degree in Gyneacology. I told Mercy I was interested to present her case to learned Gynecologists at the University Teaching Hospital once I was in School.

She was excited by this and looked forward to the day we would meet again.

Later that evening I sat in my study and digested Mercy's case. This was no case for the faint hearted.

I thought Mercy could actually be a man ensnared in a woman's body. I was almost certain she suffered from a disease resulting from failure of a male's body to respond to action of certain hormones in the body. I gave her a diagnosis of Androgen Insensitivity Syndrome (AIS). This is a disease affecting unborn male babies causing them to look like females later in life. Owing to Ambiguous Genitalia at birth, these boys are raised as girls. In the general population the disease is found 1 in 20,000 live births. Men with AIS have an appearance of normal females, despite the presence of testes. The external genitalia are female but the vagina usually ends blindly in a pouch and the uterus and uterine tubes are absent or rudimentary. At puberty there is normal development of breasts and female characteristics, but menstruation does not occur. The psychosocial orientation of a patient of AIS is female. The testes are usually in the abdomen.

In my mind, this was clearly the case with my Mercy. Owing to their complex gender state, these Males are; Medically, Legally and socially accepted as females. When a patient of AIS is discovered, usually after puberty, the abdominal Testes must be removed surgically because of a high risk for transforming into cancer

In the dead of the night, my mind wandered off into Greek Mythology; I recalled reading a story about Adonis, an extremely attractive young man who was loved by both Aphrodite and Persephone. Unfortunately, he was killed by a wild boar but Zeus ordered that he should spend the winter months in the underworld with Persephone and the summer months with Aphrodite.

Back in the day, I went to school with a gifted boy. This was an ambitious era when every adolescent hungered for a brighter future and schools delivered the most scrumptious subjects to satisfy their famished pupils. We read anything from Greek mythology to Plato's Philosophy. In contrast, kids nowadays are doomed by an Academic Apocalypse ravaging our education system.

I remembered him clearly that evening. His name was Mweene Banda. In grade eight, while the rest of us were learning Arithmetic and Civics, he was devouring Calculus, Economics and American Politics. He knew every Senator and Congressman by name and engaged any grown adult on complex theorems in Economics.

It was from this boy I first learnt about the American Revolution, Quantum theory and Vodafone revolutionary cellular net works. In order not to look like morons around this Kid, we all took to wild reading. Today, most schools lack this ravenous appetite for knowledge. This absence of competitiveness explains why everything is breaking apart; our education standards have fallen, our industries are closed, our leadership is under the spell of Pavlovian conditioning.

During the 1890s, a Russian physiologist Ivan Pavlov was looking at salivation in dogs in response to being fed, when he noticed that his dogs would begin to salivate whenever he entered the room, even when he was not bringing them food. At first this was something of a nuisance. In 1902, Pavlov started experimenting from the idea that there are some things that a dog does not need to learn. For example, dogs don't learn to salivate whenever they see food. This reflex is 'hard wired' into the dog. In behaviorist terms, it is an unconditioned response.

As the boredom of the night got the best of me, I fell asleep and dreamt. In my dream, I stood before a large audience and delivered a lecture on a confusing array of issues;

"Society as it has been known by our grandparents may be grinding to a halt around us. Many grandparents had great respect for education. Often, they encouraged the youth of their time to get an education, even when doing so, meant selling off their highly priced cattle to support their children's education.

The spirit of competitiveness in local schools needs to be restored. It is this Olympiad drive that made the once famous schools in the country; Hillcrest, David Kaunda, Mpelembe, St Mary's, etc to soar high. Oxford, Cambridge, Princeton, Yale, Harvard, UNZA, etc, owe their illustrious legacies to the competitive spirit of their scholarly Alumni.

The importance of a vibrant and competitive education system cannot be over emphasized. It is sad that many seem to be contented with the provision of a basic education to every child. In a country like ours, this should not be an option. Every child should be given the best education the nation can offer, unless that child is incapacitated by irreversibly faulty brain parenchyma. Even juvenile delinquents ought to be held in special Guantanamo Maximum Academic Prisons; where the punishment would be rigorous study of; Music, Sport, Philosophy, Art, Agriculture, Mathematics, Engineering, Law and Natural Sciences. Children are the most important resource of any nation and must be Educated to the highest standards possible.

Equal opportunity for all does not imply you now take cretins to NASA to study rocket science. Or the obtuse to train in Forensic science with Scotland Yard and send the dim witted to Harvard school of Business and Economics.

I think, like parts of the body, every man and woman has a place in this complex society and the only way to find out where each belongs is through a system of rigorous testing and examinations. Separate schools should be set to train; legs, hands, necks, fingers, eyes, ears, hearts, livers, kidneys, brains, bones, skins, etc in order to create a specialized human resource necessary to accelerate national development into the next century.

Society must revile corruption and the despicable culture of job or school placement just because you know someone. Deserving kids must be given the best places at the University even when those kids hail from Dundumwezi. The country needs them for the task ahead in the new century. The lack of money should not be a reason for falling out of school or banishment to some ridiculous trade school somewhere.

Our nation should Prioritize Education and commit resources to educate all its citizens according to their ability, genetic makeup and career interest.

Going by the Darwinian Theory; humans dominate the earth today owing to their superior brain.

Imagine if cockroaches were to bribe their way into society today and corruptly allowed to take the top spot in our civilized world; what a sight of Roaches it would be.....” I awoke the following morning feeling ill. Mercy's illness had severely affected me. For the next several weeks, I couldn't get her out of my mind.

I met Mercy six months later. My pursuit of knowledge had taken me to the School of Medicine. I had gone there to Master the Sciences of Obstetrics and Gynecology in order to solve complex health problems pounding our poor communities and ordinary citizens such as Mercy. While I was scratching my head to solve her complex illness, I found myself drawing parallels of my work and politics. I was sad to realize my country was the only patient we the people allowed even cockroaches to attend her numerous afflictions; Heart failure, Abscesses, ulcers, hernias, Bareness, Pneumonia, Poor sight, Diabetes and AIDS. It was sad to see any Jim and Jack from the streets hold high office and sit at the table tasked to solve the country's complex Economic Mayhem. Whereas medical schools were admitting only the Cream of the nation, Political Parties, and Civil Society were recruiting Savages, Barbarians and every uncivilized Scoundrels to join their ranks. It appeared to me the least respected responsibility in the nation was National Development and Governance. While Medicine required one to hold a medical degree and a valid practicing License; none was required to practice politics let alone join a political party. There were no special qualifications required for one to sit at the political round table. It was no wonder the country was still grappling with a reek of poverty in the 21st Century. While this was happening, the year elsewhere was 2005; I couldn't fathom why a forty year old country was crawling like a ten year old Trisomy 21. I was sure my country suffered from Down's syndrome. However, I chose to blame it on the chaff political parties and civil society had recruited into their ranks.

I resolved to hibernate and used the time to burry my head in my books hopping by the time of my graduation in 09, these political roaches would have been fumigated and a prosperous nation would emerge in which I would practice my Master's knowledge proudly. I eagerly looked forward to attending the FIFA World Cup in South Africa the year after my graduation.

I was hopeful those who would emerge out of hibernation in 2010 and the decades there after, would be surrounded by a prosperous nation;

governed by laws and not men. A society rid of all political scumbags, misogynists and architects of bigotry.

Mercy and I met at my new flamboyant Hospital, the University Teaching Hospital. My learned Teachers dissected her afflictions by referencing her to several syndromes they had seen in their long practice.

After weeks of deliberation, tests and scans, a decision was finally reached to operate on Mercy. I eagerly tagged along to the operating theatre to see what Pastor E's village ultra sound machine had shown in Mercy's abdomen.

In theatre, I watched the learned team rip open my poor patient's abdomen. If this had been a road construction, those unschooled imbeciles would probably sit at the table deciding which company to give the contract to. The contrast was a wonder to behold in this theatre. Only the learned Surgeons where seated at the operating table.

As I watched, I couldn't help but think politics in Africa was similar to having cleaners and potters included on the list of surgeons in the hospital. I imagined a hospital that allowed cleaners and potters to perform surgery such as the one I was watching alongside the learned surgeons. I was sure the outrage and outcry from the community demanding to close a hospital that would allow these phony surgeons from slaying millions would be deafening. Yet in politics, these communities agreed to vote for incompetent unschooled scoundrels to hold public office and execute surgeries that slay their livelihood and impede national development. Electing leaders based on populist standing is one of the root causes of Africa's endearing poverty; because had poverty been appalling, Africa would have rid itself of this malignancy long ago. Populism is another face of Dictatorships. Leaders at all levels ought to be elected like CEOs of major cooperate organizations are; to make huge profits for the citizens; on Merit for the profits at stake and never on a populist tickets. Citizens are a country's investors and share holders.

As Mercy lay on the operating table, I saw in her my country. I shuddered at the thought of her surgeons while she struggles daily to feed her children and make a profit for her investors, the citizens.

There was no womb to be found in Mercy's abdomen.

"She has no uterus," one of the surgeons spoke up.

"What is this ovoid structure here? Could it be an ovary?" another asked.

"It might as well be a Testis."

"Are you suggesting abdominal testis?"

"Boss this is clearly a case of Androgen Insensitivity Syndrome, AIS."

"How do you suggest we proceed?"

"Take out his testis of course."

"Suppose it is an Ovary? I should take a biopsy first."

"What difference does it make? How many histopathology results have we received in the past year?"

"None," the boss answered. "However this should not justify perpetuating non evidence based practices."

The two surgeons argued on how to proceed. I watched quietly with other post graduate students.

"There is no formalin in the Hospital," the theatre nurse remarked. "The biopsy will go to waste."

"That will save her Ovary from Dr Phiri's proposed management."

"The boss wins," Dr Phiri smiled and offered us a short lecture. "In the general population this disease is found 1 in 20,000 live births. Men with AIS have an appearance of normal females, despite the presence of testes.

The external genitalia are female but the vagina usually ends blindly in a pouch and the uterus and uterine tubes are absent or rudimentary. At puberty there is normal development of breasts and female characteristics, but menstruation does not occur. The psychosocial orientation of a patient of AIS is female. The testes are usually in the abdomen. Owing to their complex gender state, these Males are; Medically, Legally and socially accepted as females. When a patient of AIS is discovered, usually after puberty, the abdominal Testes must be removed surgically because of a high risk for transforming into cancer."

The two surgeons agreed to construct a vagina for Mercy and to leave her Testis/Ovary alone. After an hour and half, they constructed an eight centimeter long vagina.

It would be eight years before I ran into Mercy again. She was getting married and she wanted me to attend her wedding. The invitation took me by great surprise. Especially that I had thoroughly counseled her on her peculiar condition eight years earlier. Her Fiancé however, was delighted to proceed with the wedding despite Mercy being Male. This same sex marriage would take place in a church before an unsuspecting congregation and would probably be the first of its kind in the country.

I was deeply concerned for Mercy whether her happiness would withstand the storms lurking ahead. Just as a tree that does not produce fruit is cut down, so should economically impotent managers purporting to be running the affairs of a nation. I was aware a marriage without children rarely survives the rage of the African In-law.

48 hours

One late afternoon, I was called to the male surgical ward by a colleague asking for my opinion on a patient he had admitted two days earlier.

"Sorry doc to bother you like this," the ward Doctor started to explain when I got to the surgical ward.

"Not at all, I was just getting ready to drive out for my monotonous home. Maybe you have something interesting on your ward to take away my impending boredom," I answered.

He laughed and led me to see Mr. Hospitality.

"It is about this guy doc, his abdomen is tender and is guarding but his temperature is normal. He has not opened bowels or passed flatus for four days now. I thought of appendicitis and peritonitis but in view of normal temperature, I am entertaining a perforated ulcer, pancreatitis and intestinal obstruction as differentials. So I went ahead and ordered some x-rays to rule out intestinal obstruction."

The 26 yr old patient worked as a chef at a prestigious Rendezvous, in the hospitality industry, based in the tourist capital of Livingstone. It was famous for its exquisite continental mouth watering banquets.

What he didn't know was that some of this food he was consuming and serving had slowing burrowed its way across the wall of his stomach. A deadly ulcer had burst open emptying the contents of his gut into his belly.

Up until now my bias was on women's health and I was in-charge of Maternity and Gyneacology wards while this young enthusiastic Doctor ran Surgical Wards. That same period, I was planning on taking my membership examination with the royal college of obstetrics and gynecology. This was the same young Doctor who drugged me back into surgery at this rural hospital I was now working. I had earlier decided to abandon Surgery to concentrate on my interest in obstetrics and gynecology. However, I found myself, the further I got away from surgery, the closer I got drawn back into surgery. It is strange sometimes; the things we are cut out for are the things we try to avoid.

I recalled devoting my study to a post graduate book in my sixth year of medical school entitled 'cellular basis of surgery' as a pass time. I was now certain, the knowledge I had acquired in that book, had come back to haunt me seeking practical application.

This was my first month since reporting at this rural hospital. And the surgery I had done since arriving equaled a year's work elsewhere. I couldn't help but recall my first meeting with this hard working Foreign trained Zambian Doctor.

My surgical induction at this hospital was one for the record books. I had gone to see the young doctor for briefing before my scheduled official reporting to the hospital the following week. No sooner did I set foot at his hospital than it started raining surgical cases.

We were standing in the car park around 17 hours when a nurse appeared with some supposedly bad news; intestinal obstruction.

"Thank God I caught you before you knocked off," she said hastily.

"But I have knocked off," the young doctor protested. "What do you have?"

"Maamba Hospital has sent a case of intestinal obstruction caused by an irreducible inguinal scrotal hernia and we thought you could see before you leave," she explained.

"This is Dr Marx, he will be joining our hospital probably next week," he said introducing me to the nurse and added, "Doc, if you have time, you can come with me we check on this new admission."

Within minutes, we were hastening towards the male surgical ward. On the way, I couldn't help but think; "this is one smart beautiful young nurse. We should have more of such. Great diagnosis if she hasn't lifted it out of the referral letter. No, I am being over judgmental. She looks intelligent enough to fathom the urgency of this complication."

On the ward we found things as Nurse Einstein had described them;

$$E = MC^2$$

The young doctor turned to me and said, "Doc, I have **not** learnt to do this sort of surgery. I wish we could help this patient here. However, none of the doctors here does bowel and hernia surgery. We have to refer this patient to Livingstone."

The tone in his voice revealed humility in his heart and great willingness to learn. I was forced to reveal a part of my training I intended to conceal at this hospital; Surgery.

At my previous station, we considered this sort of surgical complication, a walk in the park. I knew exactly what to expect on the operation table.

Livingstone was 300km away from this hospital. That meant arriving at 21hrs if the Ambulance left that hour and surgery being conducted at past 23hrs.

"I can show you how to do this surgery, if you don't mind me operating before my official reporting next week," I offered getting the file from him and wrote out elaborate orders for Nurse Einstein.

"Do you do General Surgery too? I thought you are an OBG resident," He asked obviously surprised.

"It is one of the spells my last station cast on me," I replied smiling.

Nurse Einstein looked me up and down clearly unconvinced by my claim.

"Doc, I want this young nurse to come to theatre with us?' I said ignoring her disparaging gesture.

"Certainly, I am sure she has never seen this operation before," the young doctor agreed looking at Nurse Einstein squarely in the eye.

The stage was set for me to show off and shine.

In medical school we called this an opportunity to shine. I despise boasting. For me all glory belonged to God. No Doctor had power over life and Death. However that day, I really wanted to shine. I blamed my snobbish actions on Nurse Einstein.

We were in theatre by 18 hours. Several other nurses had turned up to spy on the conceited stranger masquerading as a Surgeon under the guise of seeing the operation. I took my stand on the table and hastily made a cut in the groin just above the giant swelling extending downwards and forwards into the patient's shine scrotum. I ran my incision towards the patient's pubic tubercle along his groin crease. While I did this, I expounded the architect of the inguinal canal and ran through its boundaries, contents and blood supply to important structures. The young doctor was mesmerized. Within minutes, I reached the cause of the bulge everyone had been waiting to see. Jammed dip into his inguinal canal was 45cm of small intestines that had slipped away to the scrotum and got stuck. They were black and deadly dead.

"This is necrotic bowel," I announced to the apprehensive faces in the room. I proceeded to cut off the dead bowel without contaminating the wound and meticulously rejoined the viable two ends without extending my 4 cm groin incision. I tested the point of anastomosis. It was as tight as a caned coke.

I concluded the operation by a daring technique; placing a Subcuticular suture on the potentially infected site.

The final finish astonished all the on lookers. It was as though, there was no wound at all. The young doctor looked at his nurses and remarked, "Surgery has returned to this hospital."

Had it been any other forum but medicine, I would have received a standing ovation and a tail of Paparazzo to annoy.

I had just saved a man's life by retrieving his estranged piece of bowel deep from the gallows of his scrotum and reestablished communication to replace this incapacitated segment of gut. How often do you see this on television or on our streets?

On this forum however, this wasn't news. It was simply what is expected of well trained doctors. After all, Hernia Surgery is child's play in the hands of many Surgeons. You would be stupid to expect some applause for this work, let alone remuneration for it. We serve under a socialist system where we are to love what we do and not expect remuneration for work done beyond the tour of duty; the noble profession, so we are told.

And this is the folly of being a Specialist; everything becomes Boring, it is simply expected of you to do and when you can't, you are frowned at with contempt. Fortunately for me, I could reward myself with an inner satisfaction, a sense of accomplishment for executing a surgical triumph expected only of Specialists and Consultants of surgery.

With Mr. Hospitality that afternoon, I got more than I had bargained for. This was not the sort of affliction my rural community of Macha Mission hospital catchment area suffered from. They always ate right. The last time I saw this operation was during my internship at Ndola Central Hospital. I had the wisdom to know what not to touch and without much ado, I now preferred the boredom of my home to this Deadly Ulcer.

The young doctor handed me the x-rays he had done and one look at them, I knew his stomach or duodenum had burst open. I pointed to the column of air on the right side and said, "I agree doc, it is a perforated ulcer. Good diagnosis, keep it up."

"Thank you doc," he answered. "I will prepare him for theatre right away."

"Unfortunately, I will have to pass this one. I have never done this surgery; we have to send him to Livingstone,"' I answered, pleased with my sincerity.

"That's sad; I would have loved to see this surgery," the young doctor remarked visibly sad.

"Let me call the surgeon in Livingstone to inform him about the patient," I said while the young doctor set about to organize transport to Livingstone.

I called Livingstone and the Surgeon answered as though he were waiting for my call. I hastily described our predicament.

"Doc, that's a very difficult case you have. Since it has been more than three days already, I am afraid the mortality is very high at this stage even if you where to send him here. I think try to operate on him just there. When you go in and if you find the perforation reinforce the repair site by suturing his Omentum on to it. Pull hard and downward on the stomach and retract his liver upward gently. The outcome in such cases is better when patients present within forty eight hours before multi organ dysfunction sets in from overwhelming infection. I am afraid at this stage mortality is as high as 30% even when operated on by the best surgeon on the Globe." that said, he hung up.

I looked at the young doctor and relayed the telephone conversation.

"It seems we have no choice but to do it ourselves," he said with a glow of excitement on his face.

Somehow, I loved desperate situations in surgery. They provided the ideal environment for miracles.

The patient was wheeled into theatre at 20hrs. My Assistant took his position at the table. The anesthetist intubated the patient and hooked him to the life support machine. The theatre nurse went through her instrument count with her runner. She carefully recorded the instruments on the table. She handed me the scalpel and for the first time in my life, I noticed that these instruments had some weight on them. This scalpel weighed a ton.

I opened the abdomen beginning at the sternum lower end and extended the incision to the umbilicus. Within seconds, we entered the abdominal   cavity.

We were greeted by loops of intestines coiled like rattle snakes waiting to strike. Their surface was covered by layer upon layer of sludge like material that had leaked out of his bowels and blood vessels. You could identify the constituents of his last meal. Food debris were scattered widely on his intestines. I picked up pieces of partially masticated green vegetable sections.

The Liver, in its unmistakable dark pink color, jostled in the upper portion of his abdomen under the beating of his relentless Heart. The stomach hangs below on the side like a medieval wine pouch. Without time to waste, I directed my search for the point of leak to the 'usual suspects'; the lesser curvature. However I had to pause in my haste; I needed to deliver a lecture to my apprentice. You could never be too sure in this life, the next time he would be peering down these chambers, he will be alone and keep the hopes of his patient's family; wife and children, waiting outside the operating room; that he would give their Father and husband a second chance to walk this earth by His Surgical Skill.

"Doc, let us remind ourselves of the blood supply to the duodenum, spleen and pancreas and perforations of Peptic Ulcers." I said to ease the tension on my hands. I begun to say things I had read in Gray's Anatomy while in medical school.

(Medical Jargon below [*in italics*], may skip without loss to story flow)

"This territory doc, is supplied by the *hepatic, splenic and superior mesenteric arteries; several retro duodenal branches from the right gastro-omental artery. The anterior superior pancreaticoduodenal branch of the gastro duodenal artery and the anterior inferior pancreaticoduodenal branch of the superior mesenteric artery form an arch anterior to the head of the pancreas; the posterior superior and the posterior inferior branches of the same two arteries form another arch posterior to the pancreas; the anterior and posterior inferior arteries here,* *as usual, spring from a common stem; from each arch thus formed straight vessels, called vasa recta duodeni, pass to the anterior and posterior surfaces, respectively, of the 2nd, 3rd and 4th parts of the duodenum;*

The fine network of arteries supplying the pancreas are derived from the common hepatic artery, the gastro duodenal artery, the pancreaticoduodenal arches, the splenic artery, and the superior mesenteric artery.

You must always remember never to wander too far from your mission and main objective during surgery.

Every minute ticking by, the patient's body mounts an inflammatory storm to the injury you have created.

And if you stay too long down here, the patient will not make it out alive from our third world theatre. We have no intensive care unit to seek medical recourse incase his body crushes.

So very quickly, get the job done and get out of his belly;

Now very briefly about perforation; *perforated duodenal ulcer is commoner than perforated gastric ulcer. Ulcer perforation still carries significant mortality of about 10%, particularly in the elderly and those with intercurrent disease.*

Free gas beneath the diaphragm on the erect abdominal films or chest films confirms the diagnosis in 70% of cases; as was shown by your x-rays.

Gastrografin meal maybe helpful if free gas is not present. If this turns out to be a perforated ulcer, we will repair the perforation by application of an omental patch.

For his age, I doubt it being a gastric ulcer. Perforated gastric ulcers in 15% of cases turn out to be gastric cancers.

Patients who come to the hospital late or are too ill for surgery, can be managed conservatively. You only have to insert an NGT tube for Nasogastric aspiration and IV fluids, antibiotics and antisecretory drugs."

With that I turned my attention back to the task at hand. Within minutes, we were peering down at the *Deadly Ulcer*. The defect in the duodenum was surprisingly large. It could admit the tip of my index finger. I breathed a sigh of relief and proceeded to seal of this hole in his gut.

Then I turned to the most important stage of this operation; washing his abdominal cavity to decontaminate it from the sequel of his leaking sewer line. I have never washed anyone's internal organs this thorough. We washed the surface his liver, diaphragm and all the 6m of bowels accessible to our hands. We used a total of 12 litres of warm saline to get the job satisfactorily done.

At 11pm, we emerged from the operating room looking like a pair of sanctimonious Priests. The patient was wheeled out of theatre alive and well.

Over the next days, our patient made steady recovery. He was walking by within forty eight hours under the watchful eye of his passionate wife. We allowed him to sip some plain water by within 48 hrs and he was ready to go home by day seven.

Mr. Hospitality returned to work within eight weeks of leaving hospital. He faithfully adheres to the ulcer diet we served him on discharge to this very day.

The Family

I led my team to the female surgical ward. I went to see a patient whose relatives had declined surgery. She had been on the ward for a week and the condition continued to deteriorate. I had diagnosed her with peritonitis and had planned her for immediate surgery unfortunately her mother and the rest of the family declined surgery.

When I approached her bed, I didn't like what I saw. The infection had spread into the patient's chest. Her right lung was failing to let in air. It had become like a wet sponge. Her abdomen was grossly distended. I tapped on it and it resonated like a drum. She had complicated into intestinal obstruction. A nazo- gastric tube drained copious amounts of dark green bile. She laboured with every breath she took. She was dying.

While I stood on the ward pondering what to do, the patient's father entered the ward. He had just arrived from Kasama. He had not seen his daughter since she was taken ill. He requested the nurses to allow him to see the doctors and find out for himself what he had heard on phone from his family about his daughter's illness.

"Doctor, I am the father to your patient with a swollen abdomen. I have just arrived from Kasama. Please explain to me what is wrong with my daughter," he asked.

I decided to seize this opportunity to show the father what was killing his daughter. I excused myself and told the man I needed to collect a sample to show him. When he consented, I asked the nurses and my students to place screens around the patient's bed and to give me a sixty millilitre syringe.

"Why do you want to do a speculum examination on the patient?" the nurse asked.

"Watch and learn," I answered.

I inserted a large bore needle in the space between the Uterus and the rectum through the vagina. A thick porridge like fluid filled the syringe. The students were astonished.

"This is called culdocentesis," I announced.

"OMG it is pus; it smells awful; she would have been discharged by now had she accepted the operation when she came last week. I was there when Dr Kalenga admitted her and ordered laparotomy stat however the family vehemently declined surgery," the nurse remarked closing her nose.

I walked to where the family sat on the benches next to the nurse's station. I asked Joan, one of the medical students, to hold a small dish and squeezed out the foul smelling pus for the relatives to see. They were terrified with what they saw and some looked away.

"Don't look away. You are the same people that refused the operation last week. This is what is killing your relative. Had the operation been conducted last week, she would have been discharged by now. You people never learn. Look at what your stubbornness has caused," the nurse rebuked the family. "If she dies, her blood will be on your heads. You have killed her yourselves."

"Sister," I tried to intervene.

"I am very angry with this family doc. Forgive me. One week is too long. Look at the poor woman," having rebuked the family, the nurse returned into the ward to clear the screens from the patient's bed. She was visibly angry.

"I am sorry sir, forgive the nurse. She was only expressing her concern for your daughter," I apologized for the nurse's reaction.

"She is right. We have interfered with your professional work," the father answered. "Like I said, I have just arrived; I didn't know her condition was this bad."

"Can you still operate on her in the condition she is?" a medical student asked.

"I must say, we don't accept blood, however you can go ahead and operate on her," the patient's father gave his position on blood transfusion.

I left the ward for the operating theatre. The students followed after completing thorough preparations of the patient for surgery. It was nearly half past two by now. I had not had time for Lunch. I was hungry and tired.

I arrived at the entrance after a few turns and pushed the wide double

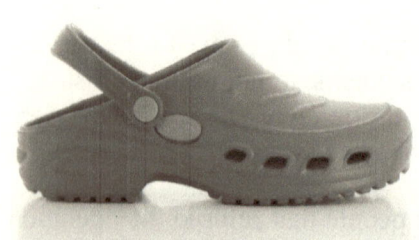

door leading into theatre. It swung open and ushered me in. The students were already in theatre waiting for me. They had taken a short cut through labour ward.

I turned right immediately into the foot wear change room and traded my shoes for the operating room Clogs. Then I walked towards the change room at the far end of the corridor where I found the anaesthetist waiting for me. He didn't look very happy to see me. I quickly primed myself for a fight.

"Doctor, why are you bringing that dying woman into my theatre? I don't think she can survive anesthesia let alone your surgery," the anaesthetist launched his attack without mincing his words. "Are you the only one who can't see that she is already dead? Why can't you just leave her alone to die peacefully? Everyone can see that she is dying. Any Jim and Jack can see that."

"Nonsense, I am not your silly Jim and Jack," I answered and almost started walking away to join my enlightened medical students. "I am not planning on opening her abdomen. Nonetheless, her family has already consented to what I intend to do. They are aware about death as a possible outcome. However, if you are uncomfortable, I will send for the other anaesthetist."

Jessica sat on a chair beside a wide work table. I walked in and sat opposite her. Joan sat on a bench just to the left of the entrance into the duty room. She rested her head in her palms. She looked beautiful as always in her blue scrubs. Felix sat with her. Johnny and George stood and leaned against an old wooden cupboard on the far right corner. It was twenty past three by now.

"How did you convince the anaesthetist into accepting this critically ill woman? You know he is difficult that one," the theatre nurse asked when she entered the duty room.

"I told him to leave if he felt uncomfortable."

"How are we going to know what is causing the pus if we don't open her abdomen?" Jessica asked.

"That is a good question. We won't know the cause. She wouldn't survive a laparotomy. I hope this would help stabilize her for definitive surgery later," I explained admiring Jessica.

"Please explain the procedure to us," Joan asked sitting upright. Her virgin breasts stood elegantly on her chest. They were kept in check by a sexy white brassiere.

Johnny looked at her chest and could see her inner aspects through the V shaped collar in her scrub. She caught his prowling eye and slowly adjusted her top with a gentle smile. He felt a tremor run up his spine, conveying his mortal nature. I felt vulnerable in the event anyone of these beautiful girls chose to seduce me. I felt defenseless in the face of my beautiful students. The patient was far safer in my hands than I was in the company of Jessica and Joan.

"The procedure will be exactly similar to what we did on the ward except, it will be on a large scale. We will make an opening into the abdomen via the vagina. We will enter posterior to the cervix into a space found between the uterus and the rectum. This space is referred to as the recto-uterine pouch or simply, pouch of Douglas. It is the lowest point in the body when a woman lies down," I explained looking at Joan. Our eyes met and she looked down. Eight years stood between us, I turned thirty one that month.

She had beautiful white eyes and lovely black eyebrows against a smooth baby face without blemishes. I thought she would have looked prettier had she chosen a career in law or Banking.

"The patient is ready," the nurse came to announce.

"Joan and Jessica, you will scrub in with me," I chose my faithful surgeons.

"No, it is our turn today. Joan and Jessica always assist you," Johnny protested.

"You are right," I answered him. "And that is why I don't change the winning team. This is not some kind of changing turns game. I have been building a team ever since I arrived here. The girls have always been with me and assisted me in many complicated cases. They have not dodged theatre like many of you boys. They have shown great eagerness to learn. I need to use the skills I have taught them in this operation. I don't want to start teaching someone raw. The patient is very sick," I defended my girls with a firm voice.

The Girls were very delighted to learn how I felt about them.

"Thank you doc for shutting the guys off, they always think dirty things about us. They think we come to theatre to see you for other things," said Joan laughing at Johnny.

"I know. Have you ever seen the homunculus of a man?" I asked.

"No," Joan answered.

"A naked woman sits on it," I answered with a grin.

They all burst out laughing. We entered operating room 2 after crossing the surgeon's scrub area.

***

The patient lay on the table barely breathing. A black oxygen mask covered her mouth and nose. The anaesthetist stood by the head end angry. I walked in with my students talking cheerfully.

It was quiet outside. The visiting hour was over and people were hurrying, returning to their various homes in family groups. The sun flew low on the western horizon. A cold breeze swept across the hospital. Dusk was upon the small town of Mbala. As they walked back to their homes, some Families discussed this patient. It was clear, as the anesthetist had observed, even to lay people, the patient was dying.

The anesthetist was angry because I had taken a hopeless case to theatre.

The nurse positioned her instruments table to my right. I sat on a stool at the foot end of the operating table. Joan stood closely to my left. Her waist rubbed against my left shoulder. We stood between the patient's legs which were placed on special supports and strapped at the knees.

"This is called the lithotomy position," I explained.

"Like they do in labour ward," Joan remarked.

"That is correct Dr Joan," I agreed looking up at Joan. She was a tall girl and towered gracefully above my head. "Lithotomy is a medical term referring to a common position for surgical procedures and medical examinations involving the pelvis and lower abdomen, as well as a

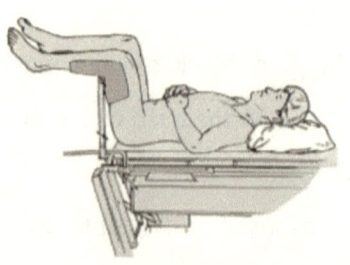

common position for childbirth like Joan said. The lithotomy position involves the positioning of an individual's feet above or at the same level as the hips, often in stirrups, with the perineum positioned at the edge of the examination table or operating table as in our case here."

"It is a very bad position when it is done with a fully conscious person," Jessica observed. She was scrubbed in and stood on the patient's right waiting for my instructions.

"You are right. Actually patients have reported feeling a loss of control and increased sense of vulnerability when examined in the lithotomy position because they cannot see the area being examined. Other, equally effective positions have been suggested for examinations of conscious patients," I agreed.

"That is better, I would cry on you if you placed me in this position Dr Marximillian," said Joan laughing and stealing a glance at me.

"I am sure he wouldn't want to do it under such conditions too," the anaesthetist remarked joining the conversation.

"Sir, she is only a child," the theatre nurse came to Joan's rescue. Everyone burst out laughing.

"It is good to have you back sir. I am sorry about our little fight earlier. You know I enjoy working with you," I said looking across at the anaesthetist.

"You are welcome doc. I was wrong," he answered.

"Now back to Dr Joan's position," I paused for a reaction from my beautiful assistants.

"No Dr Marx, I fear this position. You can kill someone," she remarked laughing.

"Don't worry, our patient won't die," I assured her. "References to this position have been found in some of the oldest known medical documents including versions of the Hippocratic Oath. The position is named after the ancient surgical procedure for removing Kidney stones and bladder stones via this route, the perineum. The position is perhaps most recognizable as the 'often used' position for childbirth: the patient is laid on the back with knees bent, positioned above the hips, and spread apart through the use of stirrups. The position is frequently used and has many obvious benefits from the doctor's perspective."

I paused to allow for a reaction from the house.

"Doc, it also has many domestic benefits," the anaesthetist remarked.

"Dr Joan and Dr Jessica here are not yet 19. You will confuse them," I warned the anaesthetist as I rose from my stool.

"That is not true sir. We are big girls. We'll turn 23 next month," Jessica protested.

"Then I will continue with my lecture; 'benefits of the Lithotomy position', uncensored," I smiled. "Most notably the position provides good visual and physical access to the Perineal region and most important, to the vagina. The position is used for procedures ranging from simple pelvic exams, like we did on the ward, to complex surgeries like the one we are performing right now. However, new observations and scientific findings, combined with a greater sensitivity to patient needs have raised awareness of the physical and psychological risks the position may pose for prolonged surgical procedures, pelvic examinations, and, most notably, childbirth. A Cochrane Review found that the lithotomy position may not be the ideal position for child birth, noting that while it makes care easier for midwives and doctors by placing the patient in an easily accessible position, it is often harder on birthing mothers as use of the lithotomy position can narrow the birth canal by up to a third. In lieu of the lithotomy position, the Cochrane Review recommended birthing mothers make informed choices about birthing positions and find the position that is most comfortable for them."

"It is the same in the home, there are now many positions to choose from," the anaesthetist continued with his domestic discourse. "Actually doc, these young girls nowadays, know sophisticated positions that would make your eyes fill up with a torrent of tears and easily kill you from a heart attack."

The theatre nurse burst out laughing. The boys joined in laughing on top of their voices.

"Leave my doctors alone. These are angels. They do not know of any such positions you are talking about," I defended my lovely assistants with a firm voice. However a grin on my face gave me away.

By now, the runner had brought twenty litters of saline and another twenty litters of distilled water from the laboratory. I proceeded to open the posterior fornix and introduced two large drainage tubes. Copious amounts of foul smelling pus came gushing out.

Felix turned on the suction machine and filled three litres of brownish white pus within ten minutes. I passed one drainage tube to Jessica and instructed her to pour saline through the tube at will. George, who had been very quiet all this while, assisted Jessica on the right side. I passed the second tube to Kaoma and her assistant, Kaluba.

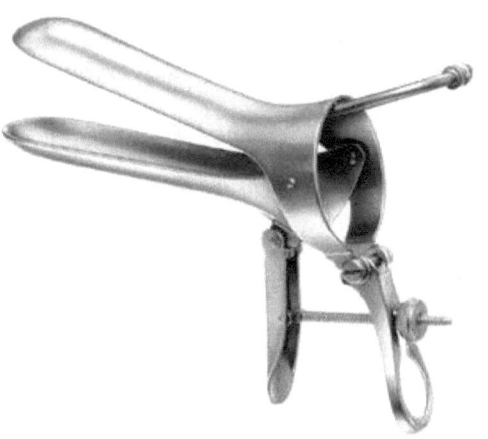

Joan assisted me at the perineum. Her responsibilities included holding the irrigation tubes in the pouch of Douglas and keeping the vagina open with a Sims speculum.

"Poor woman, she is rotten inside. If she survives, she should thank God you came. We would not have touched her if it weren't for you. You are a brave man Dr Marximillian, you really are," said the anaesthetist looking at me.

I was busy working between the patient's legs.

"You see why I needed all of you here. Where are the others, the priest and Shifu? Were they not with you in the duty room?" I asked.

"They went back to the hostels. They thought you only wanted Joan and Jessica," Kaluba answered.

"That is the reason I do not teach surgery to lazy students. These are dangerous skills to place in the hands of malingerers," I stood up and let Joan continue guiding the abdominal irrigation.

After several litters of saline, the job was finally done. The patient's abdomen flattened out and her breathing showed some remarkable improvements. I was pleased with the work my team had done. I left the hospital at 10pm.

A Stitch in Time

I checked my 'to do list' ....a visit to Moto Moto Museum was next. I was much more interested to check out the Traditional Medicines section. I couldn't wait to lay my hands on some raw materials for testing in my home based laboratory. I had heard about Akamyanshinge, a potent Aphrodisiac for treating impotence in men and that could arouse incredible libido in both sexes. I had also heard about Musengele, a potent love charm. I also hoped to lay my hands on Kaselelele, a potent traditional Oxytocic drug used to accelerate labour in home deliveries and probably responsible for some of the uterine raptures I had attended at the Local Hospital.

The Moto Moto Museum was a Must see. I couldn't wait to experiment with a pinch. As I thought these things, my phone rang. It was the coverage nurse. There was an emergency at the hospital and they wanted me urgently.

"Doc, I have a woman with Hb 6g/dl. She has APH at term. I can't appreciate the foetal heart beat. She is only a tip of finger and she is 'O' minus. There is no blood in the hospital. I am considering referring her," the doctor on call explained.

"Let me come over," I replied.

The emergency vehicle arrived shortly. It was 11 pm in Mbala. We drove for the hospital immediately. The driver was counting on me to call off the referral to Kasama, and save him 400 km night driving. We drove in the dark silently. It was late and I was tired. I summoned my mind to recall all what I knew about APH.

Now APH is Antepartum Haemorrhage or heavy bleeding before delivery. This call brought a deluge of nostalgic memories of my days as an OBGY Resident. The Landcruiser bounced and jerked on the treacherous bumpy gravel road to the Hospital. It was dark all around except for the poor light from the head lumps and tail lights of the old cruiser. It was cold inside the cruiser. Its wipers worked frantically to keep an unrelenting drizzle over Mbala off its cracked windscreen. Visibility was poor. I was glad it was only a short drive to the hospital.

On arrival at the hospital, I rushed to the Maternity ward through the dark corridors. I found the Doctor on call anxiously waiting for me as were several midwives on duty that cold Mbala night. My students had gone to the ward too when news about this emergency reached them.

"Hi guys," I greeted the students in my usual calm temperament. "What do you have doc?"

"I think we should just refer this woman doc," the exhausted doctor on call gave his opinion. He had surrendered.

"Do you think she has better chance of survival if you refer her than here? Remember Kasama is not next door," I challenged the exhausted doctor.

"Her Hb is 6g/dl and we have no blood in the hospital," a midwife came to the rescue of the doctor.

I turned to my students and begun to teach.

"Obstetric haemorrhage remains one of the major causes of maternal death in developing countries. The causes of APH include; Placenta previa, Placental abruption and local causes. It is not uncommon to fail to identify a cause of APH, when it is then described as 'unexplained APH'.

"I was thinking she has a ruptured uterus or placenta previa," the doctor on call tried to explain.

"No doc, this is Placental abruption," I explained walking over to examine his patient.

"How can you tell placenta previa from placenta abruption," O'Neil asked.

"Usually placenta previa causes painless bleeding," Joan answered.

"That is very correct Dr Joan," I agreed. "Abruptio placentae is defined as the premature separation of a normally positioned placenta from the wall of the uterus, usually after 20 weeks of pregnancy. Patients with Abruptio placentae, also called placental abruption, typically present with vaginal bleeding, painful uterine contractions, and fetal distress or death like in our case here."

While I taught, I was worried the patient might develop the most feared complication of all; couvelaire's uterus. This was my last week in Mbala and the last thing I needed was a patient dying on the operating table. I knew everyone would forget all the good surgeries I had performed and only remember this one poor outcome. I stood for a while and pondered the words of the doctor on call to refer the patient to die on the way to Kasama. I was almost certain; this was a conspiracy against the good work I had done. The temptation to refer the patient weighed heavily on my mind.

"Are you going to operate with Hb of 6 or allow her to deliver vaginally since the baby is dead?" Jessica asked looking very worried and concerned for the poor patient.

"The cervix is only admitting a tip of finger. Vaginal delivery is the best choice with a non viable fetus. However, our patient will exsanguinate before we could achieve that. Even then, she would be at risk of PPH from couvelaire's uterus. And complicate into or die from Disseminated Intravascular Coagulopathy and Acute Renal Failure," I laid out my worst case scenario.

"What is Couvelaire's uterus and DIC?" Joan asked with an perplexed look on her face.

"Couvelaire's uterus my dear, also known as uteroplacental apoplexy, is a life threatening condition in which loosing of the placenta, Abruptio placentae, causes bleeding that penetrates into the uterine muscles, the myometrium, forcing its way into the peritoneal cavity. The treatment involves immediate evacuation of the uterus and stimulating uterine contractions with intravenous oxytocin; Hysterectomy, the removal of the uterus, may be needed in some cases," I explained to my stunned team. "DIC is a serious disorder in which the proteins that control blood clotting become over active.

"Hysterectomy with Hb of 6; doc let us just refer this patient to Kasama. She will die on us. I don't want her blood on my hands," the doctor on call reiterated his call for referral.

"I think Dr Okocha is right. Let us just refer her. We have no blood here," a Midwife answered taking Dr Okocha side.

"Those in favour of referral raise your hands," Mr. Okocha and the midwife raised their hands. "If Medicine was a democracy, we would have settled this by a show of hands. Fortunately it is not. This is why I think our current voting system, one man one vote, is foolish; You and I have the same voting power as a retarded unschooled bastard who spends his day drinking at a street corner somewhere. I think each of your votes should equal a thousand votes."

"Your vote Dr Marximillian should equal a million votes," said Joan smiling at me.

"I couldn't agree with you more my love," I answered smiling warmly. "I called Kasama on my way here. They have no blood. It would be tantamount to immorality to send this patient a long way off, only to die on the way to Kasama. This might be her only window of survival. If she must die by my hand, so be it. Sister, prepare this patient for surgery; we are going in. Girls, you will be my assistant surgeons.

"Doc, this patient was in shock when I was called. Her uterus was not contracting that is why I thought she had placenta previa. She may truly have couvelaire's uterus. The uterus won't contract. You may be faced with a real hysterectomy with an Hb of 6. I have never seen anyone perform a hysterectomy under these circumstances. I have a feeling this is not likely to turn out right," Dr Okocha spelt out his consternation.

"May be this is her appointed time to die. Why can't you just leave her alone to die peacefully? I have a bad feeling about this too," the midwife echoed Dr Okocha's premonition.

"I am a scientist. I do not use feelings. I make scientific decisions," I put my foot down.

Everyone was quiet. The students brought the theatre trolley. The anesthetist watched quietly at a distance. He knew I wouldn't walk away from the patient even when her chances of survival were bleak.

(Medical Jargon below [*in italics*], may skip without loss to story flow)

"For my baby doctors, I want to tell you a little bit about the pathophysiology of this killer condition. Like I said earlier; *Couvelaire's uterus is a phenomenon wherein the retro-placental blood may penetrate through the thickness of the wall of the uterus into the peritoneal cavity. This may occur after Abruptio placentae. The hemorrhage that gets into the deciduas basalis ultimately splits the decidua, and the hematoma may remain within the decidua or may extravasate into the myometrium. The myometrium becomes weakened and may rupture due to the increase in intrauterine pressure associated with uterine contractions. Whereas, Disseminated Intravascular Coagulopathy is characterized by systemic activation of blood coagulation, which results in generation of and deposition of fibrin, leading to micro vascular thrombi in various organs and contributing to multiple organ dysfunction syndrome. Consumption and subsequent exhaustion of clotting factors or coagulation proteins and platelets, from ongoing activation of coagulation, may induce severe bleeding. Therefore, we define DIC as an acquired syndrome characterized by the intravascular activation of coagulation with loss of localization arising from different causes.*"

"This patient is already showing signs of DIC and he insists on going ahead with surgery," Dr Okocha whispered to the midwife. I overheard their gossip.

"I heard that," I answered. "God did not send me here to slaughter his people. He promised to save everyone I touched. I believe he is with us right now. This is not a feeling. It is scientifically true. I have evidence he has been with me since I came here as he has been with me in my practice back in my hospital. Do you know where David drew the courage to slay the giant?"

"From God," Jessica answered.

"It is written in 1 Samuel 17:32-37," I decided to quote my favourite scriptures;

David said to Saul, "Let no one lose heart on account of this Philistine; your servant will go and fight him."

Saul replied, "You are not able to go out against this philistine and fight him; you are only a boy and he has been a warrior from his youth."

But David said to Saul, "Your servant has been keeping his father's sheep. When a lion or bear came and carried off a sheep from the flock, I went after it, struck it and rescued the sheep from its mouth. When it turned on me, I seized it by its hair, struck it and killed it. Your servant has killed both the lion and the bear; this uncircumcised Philistine will be like one of them, because he has defied the armies of the living God. The LORD who rescued me from the paw of the lion and the paw of the bear will rescue me from the hand of this Philistine."

The team arrived in theatre. The patient was laid on the table. I instructed my young doctors to scrub in and assist me.

"No, I will assist," Dr Okocha protested. "I have heard about your bullet speed surgeries. I would like to witness one with my own naked eyes."

"Be my guest doubting Thomas," I replied and grinned at the girls.

Dr Okocha and I scrubbed in the usual way. We then approached the theatre nurse on her instruments table. She gowned us in the usual elaborate etiquette of the operating theatre. Soon we were standing on the operating table ready to start the surgery. Doubt was written all over Dr Okocha's face. I chose to ignore his disparaging facial expressions.

I proceeded to open the patient's abdomen using a lower bikini line incision. Within seconds I delivered the dead baby before Dr Okocha could say Couvelaire's uterus. I passed it to the equally thunderstruck midwife still attached to its placenta. I then turned my attention to the uterus as Dr Okocha's hands trembled continuously. I was certain my assistant surgeon would suffer a syncope attack and fall to the ground.

"Are you ok doc?" I asked him.

"You are a magician doc," he answered fumbling for words. "I have never witness such speed in my entire practice of medicine. I thought people were exaggerating when they talked about you. Now I have seen for myself. You are incredible doc."

While Dr Okocha stood dazed by the rapidly changing operating techniques he was witnessing, I had completed detaching the uterus from its upper attachments and pedicles. I spared both ovaries after examining them meticulously. The patient hardly bled.

"Where did you learn all this," the astonished Dr Okocha asked. "I should have known. I wouldn't have talked about that referral. I would have just sent for you immediately."

"I learnt it as a shepherd boy tending my sheep in remote local brown pastures," I replied placing clamps on utero- sacral ligaments. "We need to suture the vaginal vault to these ligaments to prevent prolapse in the future."

"Hysterectomy in twelve minutes, I must be dreaming," Dr Okocha remarked utterly flabbergasted.

"It is not a dream doc," the anesthetist answered him. "This is why I have always been telling you to tag along and learn before this man returns to his hospital. This is how he works. It does appear like magic, doesn't it?"

"I take off my hat for you," said Dr Okocha bowing down.

"No doc, I don't deserve that," I protested. "This is simple surgery which anyone can learn with time."

Meantime, Joan, Jessica and Serena followed the midwife to take a close look at the dead baby. The boys, Johnny, O'Neil and Shifu took Couvelaire's uterus to the sluice room for closer examination. By now, I had placed five sutures on the patient's abdomen and the theatre nurse was preparing a dressing for the wound. The anesthetist instituted his steps for reversal of his patient from anesthesia. It was a successful operation. One still talked about at Abercorn Central Hospital to this very day.

Joshua

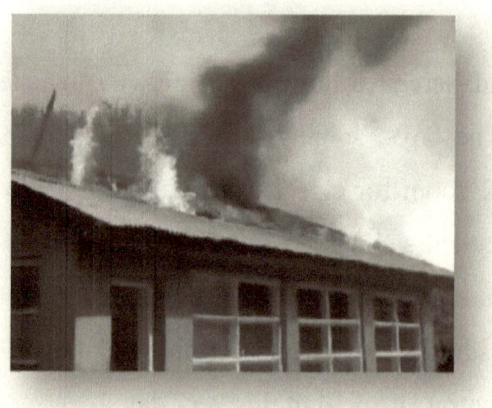

Out of a clear blue sky, on a hot July afternoon, unimaginable horror came plummeting down and struck the safest place on earth I called my home. The inferno roared and devoured everything in its path leaving a trail of indescribable devastation and shock. In the twinkling of an eye, the ten year labour of my hand was gone.

I arrived at the scene like a man awaking from a dream within a dream. Despicable scenes of shock awaited me. What once was my house, just earlier that day, became a raging furnace. I watched, helplessly, the incineration of my assets acquired over a period of Ten years by the Labors of my hand. The rising billows of smoke could be seen for miles away hauling testimony to the apocalypse that hit the house I called Home sweet home just a few hours earlier. My children, John and Jay, aged 3 and 7 respectively, watched the inferno gruesomely maul their house scattered among the multitude of people that was drawn to the scene. Here a new danger hung over their heads from flying debris and possible stampede in an event of an explosion or any terror that would send the crowd scampering.

I struggled to awake but the nightmare gripped me by the neck forcing me to look on in total bewilderment. I kicked and punched my body hoping to awake but remained incarcerated by this horror.

I was totally confused. I ran around the house dreading the worst and only short of running into the burning house to see for myself the nightmare awaiting me.

But just then, I heard two small voices I recognized to be those of my two boys crying.

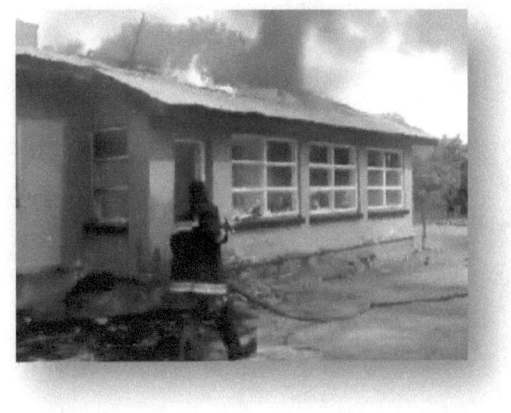

"Dad, dad! my toys are burnt. My Mini Cooper and Teddy are burning in the fire," John was crying; mourning the loss of his favorite toys.

"Dad, dad; my play station and my bicycle are burnt. My black board and my duster are burning in the house," Jay was calling.

"Where is your Mother? Where is the baby? Where is Matildah?" I asked my poor boys a barrage of questions which only an adult ought to be asked. I couldn't contain the thought that they might be trapped inside the furnace before my eyes. I dreaded running into an adult who might just confirm my worst fear. My Wife, my three week old son, my 11 year old daughter and our maid remained to be accounted for. I felt my eyes hurt; my tear glands could no longer contain the tsunami of tears building up inside their walls and soon burst open. I struggled to restrain myself. My voice quivered waiting to let out a loud cry.

The crowd merely watched; no one approached me to steady my spinning head. I was sure they knew something I didn't and that they couldn't find someone to break the bad news to me. So I simply held on to my two boys, fighting my tears back; not wanting to be seen crying by them.

Where was their dad to wrestle and quench this inferno? Where was their dad to gather his children and family to safety? Where was their dad when they needed him the most?

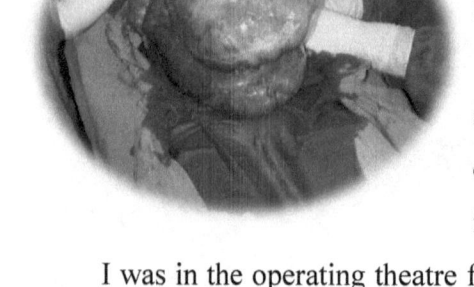

Where was their Dad to rescue their earthly possessions and future inheritance?

Their dad had been busy at work saving patients' lives while his children narrowly escaped the raging inferno to cheat death.

I was in the operating theatre faced with one of the worst intestinal obstruction I have ever seen in a female patient. Her abdomen had been so distended that it looked like she would explode at any moment. She had a Sigmoid Volvulus of more than a week and precariously very ill.

The picture above shows the findings inside her abdomen.

Earlier that day, I left home like on any other ordinary day; I bade good bye to my wife and dropped the kids at school;

"Honey, have a great day at home," I said.

"You too, have fun in theater. Wish I could join you. Should I keep lunch for you?" she asked while giving my tie a final touch.

"Prepare something nice. Some sausage or roast chicken, I'll invite the medical students over for lunch," I whispered in her ear bending to kiss her goodbye and made for the car park.

…The kids were already in the car and as usual fighting for seats.

"Have you done your homework guys?" I asked before hitting the ignition.

"Yes, we have. Mine was easy," Jay answered.

"You know the rule," I reminded them.

"Dad has to see the books before starting off," Jay answered.

"Home work done, book left at home is homework not done," I sung them my morning anthem and reflected on my typical day when I was their age.

I recalled one cold June morning, waking up my own dad to cut for me 100 'finger long' sticks from the mulberry trees that formed the fence of our house. The teacher wanted to introduce some advanced mathematics and he wanted each 2nd grader armed with some counting sticks. Good old Dad cut the sticks with lots of apprehension. He knew kids of my kind had better ideas for counting than carrying stacks of sticks. The sticks never saw the inside of my class room. "How time flies," I thought to myself.

Satisfied, they remembered to carry their homework, I hit the ignition to awake the 710 horses compressed in my V8 engine made in Germany. Life was good.

I dropped the kids at school and looked forward to a great time in the operating theater.

It was Thursday, my Elective Surgery day at the Hospital. I had a number of surgeries lined up and medical students to teach. I had thoroughly checked my patients for fitness to undergo surgery the previous day. All were fit except one. What could honestly go wrong apart from one; this one patient had been admitted at dawn for intestinal obstruction and I planned to start with her. It was a perfect day to be alive and to be doing what I loved most; the work given to me by Yahweh. The work I called passion of care.

Once at the hospital, I steered my horses into the car park and killed the Engine. Three weeks earlier, I had been recalled from my vacation leave to help out at the hospital owing to a shortage of medical officers that had suddenly befallen the hospital. I was still cranking myself to get in full swing for work and on this day, I had finally found my footing and was looking forward to having a great time in the O.R.

The anesthetist was already in theatre, but looked somewhat unhappy. I knew he was allergic to length theatre lists. That morning list was very long indeed and he was visibly upset by it.

"Doc, are you aware about this list. And if you start teaching, we won't finish," he complained while following me to the change room.

"How many patients have been added? I asked pretending to be ignorant about the list.

"14!" he screamed. "Please sir, do something about it. I need to rush into town to look for some money, my children are starving."

"By the way, Good morning Mr. Tajo,"

"I am not well doctor. How are you?" he answered. "This list has made me ill."

"I am very well Mr. Tajo. Everyone is well at home and in good health," I responded to easy him up while searching for the perfect line to address his concerns.

Mr. Tajo was the only anesthetist at this hospital and was on call 24/7. He was going through a burn out. I understood him perfectly well. He had a big family that had grown over the years however his salary had remained meager and his pay slip heavily littered by Shylocks in town. He had given his whole heart to the profession he loved but the system was not looking after him well.

"I will look at the list Mr. Tajo," I answered calmly. "How much are you looking for sir? I would be glad to assist."

Just that sentence appeared to have taken a load off his shoulders. With Mr. Tajo cooled down, I entered theatre and it was business as usual in the O.R. The woman afflicted by intestinal obstruction was wheeled into theater and the team was soon busy around her like worker ants attending the queen. Each one engrossed in their special area of training and skill; Potters, runners, theatre nurses, Mr. Tajo and Surgeon blending like notes of a symphony in a master's hand. This was my favorite moment; watching the team coordinating professionally to save the life of another human being, without regard to social economic status, Tribe or color of the patient. On this operating table, all patients were equal.

While reflecting on Professionalism; I recalled a close encounter a friend of mine had with a Judge at a local High Court in his town; He had gone to have his daughter's travel documents Authenticated. While he sat at the reception waiting to be attended, a Judge walked into the foyer where he sat; the receptionist, seeing that my friend had waited for such a long time, requested the judge whether he could help and authenticate the papers.....

"Excuse me sir, could you please assist this man, he has been waiting for a long time...." the receptionist made a request.

The Judge was brought to a sudden halt in his haste, and answered....; "I am a Judge.... I am employed to Judge and writing reports to ministers and permanent secretaries.... I don't do that sort of work you are asking me to do. Go and find a clerk to do that.... And if you will excuse me, I am rushing into court right now.... I am going to Judge... I am going to pass Judgment... this is what I do... I Judge."

Having said this, the judge reached for his robs, wore them and majestically strode to his courtroom...

Instead of being angry at such un-Zambian rejection, my friend was very happy and remarked... "That's my man. He knows his job." He later told me, if he had the opportunity, he would have loved to shake the judge's hand because this judge was truly a professional.

Mr. Tajo gave his anesthetic gear one final check and proceeded to hook the patient to his machines. I was afraid he would just say; this or the other was missing and so couldn't proceed. It is very important to take care of the Anesthetist; he is a crucial ingredient for a good outcome at Major Surgery. Whilst Mr. Tajo gave his machines a thorough last minute check; I delivered a brief lecture to my students;

"Volvulus occurs when an air-filled segment of colon twists about its mesentery. The sigmoid colon is involved in up to 70% of cases. Other Volvulus that can occur involves the ceacum in less than 20% of cases. The transverse colon is another portion of gut prone to Volvulus."

.....Satisfied with the oxygen saturation and good air entry in both lungs and the Blood Pressure; Mr. Tajo nodded I could go ahead and start. I hesitated a moment still wanting to lecture; "this patient has raised white blood cell count and a high fever; these are heralds of gangrenous bowel."

No sooner did we open up the woman's abdomen than my diagnosis was confirmed. It was a gangrenous sigmoid colon. This is to say; her last portion of large intestine that joins the rectum was rotten. It had twisted as defined; on its mesentery. The mesentery is a loose extension of special skin that covers   intestines and anchors bowels to the posterior abdominal wall. The mesentery also transmits a vast network of blood vessels to and fro the intestines. When the sigmoid twists, these blood vessels twist too; cutting off blood supply to intestines resulting into ischemia and without urgent surgical intervention, this complicates into gangrene; The case in point. I straightened up and ventured to lecture on;

(Medical Jargon below [*in italics*], may skip without loss to story flow)

"Clinical evidence of gangrene or perforation mandates immediate surgical exploration without attempt at endoscopic decompression. Similarly, the presence of necrotic mucosa, ulceration, or dark blood seen on endoscopy examination suggests strangulation and is an indication for operation. If dead bowel is present at laparatomy as in this operation you are witnessing on this beautiful day, the 28th of July, a sigmoid colectomy with end colostomy may be the safest operation to perform. This is known as Hartmann's procedure. It was first described by a French Surgeon, Henri Albert Hartmann in 1921."

Without much ado, I resigned my mind to Hartmann's operation, a three to four hour operation in my untrained hands. The operation was a success. And Mr. Tajo was very happy, the operation took us only an hour and twenty minutes by his watch. I thanked him and headed for the change room to get some refreshments. My back that was hurting. .I looked at Mr.

Tajo's List. It stated; Inguinal scrotal hernia, skin graft, Hysterectomy for Fibroids, ICD insertion, Below knew Amputation, Elective Caesarean Section in three previous Caesar, Rectal Vaginal Fistula repair, ...

While I gazed at the List, my phone rang.

"Doc, urgently get home, there is a problem..." the voice spoke with a cold tone and immediately hung up.

I held my phone expecting more detail. It went cold. Who was this that knew of a problem at my house before me the owner of the house knew anything about it. I refused to believe him. But there was something in his voice that beckoned me to do as he said.

I left theatre immediately without alarming the Team. I reached for my horses in the car park and raced home. On the way, I pondered through a list of things I thought could go wrong on a bright July afternoon.

What I found equaled my wildest guess; "a plane crashing into my house."

Indescribable scenes of Hell itself awaited me: My house was on fire; I ran into the yard dreading to smell Jet Fuel and bumping into someone that could just confirm my worst fear;

An angry inferno roared and blazed from the roof of the house. The flames rose several meters high into the sky like a killer forest fire; the accompanying thick fumes of black smoke blackened the blue sky above. The flames could be seen through all the windows of the house. They shattered through the glass and were extending their grip, in rapid succession of violent flaming waves, to anyone daring to draw near. A great multitude of people stood solemnly at a distance and watched helplessly. I scanned the premises swiftly for furniture that had signs of rescue from the house. There was none. To worsen it all; the front and lounge inner exit doors were still shut. I couldn't see any signs of escape.

I knew immediately what ever happened, hit the house very quickly. It did not give the people present any chance to evacuate anything. This analysis increased my nightmare a 100fold for the people who were in the house. I refused to accept my family could be trapped inside the furnace blazing before my eyes.

I circled the house several times, accompanied by my faithful dogs, Major, a black bull mastiff and Spike, a Rottweiler. I was hoping to hear a faint voice calling for help, but none came. At the rear of the house, a small group had managed to break through the burglar bars to the nursery and was rescuing a few possessions. I ran to the front again looking out for signs of life in the house. A sense of loss so intense that it immediately dried my mouth and throat struck me; my legs started to give way and my head started spinning: I knew I wouldn't be able to stand very long, I was about to pass out.

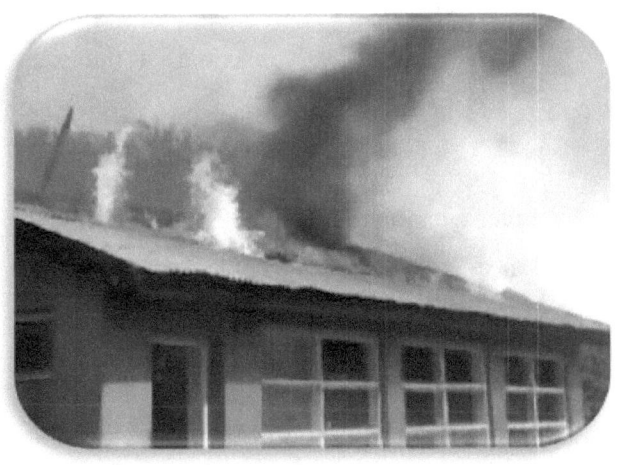

In anticipation of my impending syncope

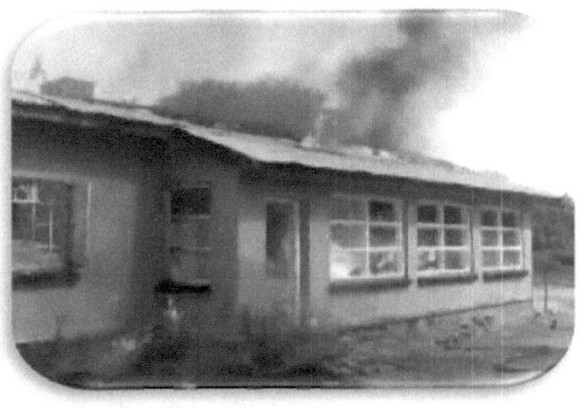

attack, I retreated backwards to join the crowd hoping to find someone or something I could clutch to for support. I was rapidly losing balance and I knew consciousness would soon follow; just then I heard two voices I recognized to be those of my children. Momentarily, I felt strength return into my body however, my eyes were like a watering cane by now. A deluge of tears blinded my sight. I could not remember the last time my face let out a tear; let alone this much. I was overwhelmed by intense feelings of loss. I could no longer compute the appropriate emotion to display to those around me. For a moment I surrendered myself to be taken over by untamed basic human instincts; I wept.

When I cleared my eyes to stare at the house again, a man I vaguely recognized to be Mr. Five, in his mid-thirties, stood in my view. Five was my neighbor…

"Five, what happened here?" I asked him.

"I was standing at the window and I saw your child playing with matches on the mattress. While I was looking at the girl, the mattress caught fire. I ran into the house to put off the fire but it had grown very big while I was still rescuing the madam and it torched the roof," he answered bluntly.

"A mattress…!" I exclaimed in shock. 'And you couldn't stop a child playing with matches. You couldn't put off a burning mattress. Your story sucks and reeks. You are the one that burnt this house and you ought to be locked up for Arson," I reacted angrily and minted out charges on him caring less on the correct term for this crime.

With the smoking gun cast into my house, I searched, feverishly, for the remaining members of my household. Two nurses from a local private surgery came over to where I was standing and said my wife and three week old son had been evacuated to their surgery.

"Do you have any news about my daughter Latildah and our house keeper Latricia?' I asked fearing to hear ghastly news. ....The presence of these nurses worsened my apprehension for grisly news. I was sure they had been sent to break it to me. And break it they did; only it was good, At least for the moment.

"As far as we know, we have not received any casualties from the house," one of the nurses spoke up.

"Your wife and baby are at the surgery. She is in a state of shock. She has no physical injuries or signs of smoke inhalation. The baby is fine too and we left him breastfeeding," the other nurse added.

While I was assimilating their presentation; my wife appeared followed by three women I could not identify. She was crying and visibly shaken. They were preventing her to go back to the house.

"She shouldn't be here, this is very traumatic for her; take her back to the surgery," one of the nurses advised the women.

"Leave me alone, I want my children, I have come to look for my children," she protested. "Where is Jo? Where is Latildah? Where is Jay?"

Just then, Latildah and Latricia our house keeper emerged from among the crowd to join us. They were visibly terrified too. The two boys had been taken to the neighbors for refuge. Relief rained on me like a piece of parched desert land. No life had been lost. But the accusing finger pointed harshly at my family.

I immediately made the decision to take my family to the police station to give statements. I decided I would hear their story at the police station. I didn't want them to present a rehearsed tale. The hunt for the Smoking gun was on; a deluge of questions poured through my mind as I raced for the police station; what burnt the house? How did the fire start?

What caused the fire? What burnt the house? What did the people in the house see?

We were received by a cold hearted sergeant at the police station. He had no emotion on his face and his voice was military harsh.

My wife was brought to the stand and the sergeant grilled her without empathy. I realized he was trained this way, to treat everyone guilty till proven innocent. Or was it; innocent till proven guilty. Things don't work that way during interrogations...... You are the suspect. Therefore you are the guilty one till proven innocent. I watched helplessly as my poor wife was battered with incriminating questions while holding the baby to her breast.

"Were you ironing cloths before the fire started?" the sergeant spat out his first question.

"No! I wasn't ironing," she answered.

"Who was ironing then? Who left the iron on?" the dim witted sergeant pressed on.

"No one and no iron was on," she answered surprised at the questions she was being asked.

"Then what were you cooking that burnt the house?" the sergeant's incriminating questions persisted.

"We had just finished having Lunch and I was at the dining table winding up, the stove was off, the kids were playing outside. The baby was in his nursery sleeping," she replied.

"Which room had petrol?" the Sergeant cut in.

"We don't keep petrol," she replied getting angry. "If you must know, we refuel our vehicles at the service station like all civilized people of this town."

"Where do you keep it then," the sergeant probed further.

"Go ask the Filling station. We don't keep petrol anywhere!' retorted my wife angry this time. "Doesn't this station have any sane sergeants to take my statement? I see that you are drunk."

"How did you burn the House and why did you burn it?" the Sergeant probed further looking at her squarely in the eye.

"We did not burn the house; I told you we had just finishing having lunch about 13:45, everything happened very fast," she answered calmly and looking back at him.

"Then tell us what happened," continued the sergeant as cold as a frog.

"I don't know what happened. I was at the dining table winding up. Then I began to smell something like burning paper in the house. I asked the maid whether there was anyone burning paper in the house…...."

"Where was the maid?" the sergeant cut in.

"She was sweeping the space between the kitchen and the dining room," she continued.

The sergeant nodded and let her continue….

"The maid told me, there was no one burning paper in the house. She further reminded that I shouldn't be having a bad sense of smell since I had delivered now. But I was so sure something was burning. So I stood up to take a look. When I opened the door from the kitchen leading to the bedrooms, I suddenly realized this smell could be coming from the nursery; I ran to the bedroom where my baby was; screaming, my baby! my baby!"

"Where was the maid at that point?" the sergeant asked.

"I don't know. I ran to pick my baby terrified I would find he had burnt. I was afraid his room might be on fire. We keep the heater on in his room to keep the baby warm. However when I got to the room, it was clear and the heater was off. The TV was on. So I picked my baby and quickly left the room holding the baby in my hands and started running. In the corridor, I was met by Mr. Five. Just then he opened a door on his right. Thick hot black fumes of smoke came gushing out into the corridor where we stood facing each other. These hot fumes blocked me from crossing over to the side he was standing. He was standing a few steps clear from the gushing fumes of hot smoke. At that pointing, he started calling to ran and cross over to where he stood. However, I couldn't the smoke was too hot. I was afraid I might burn. Without warning, it became dark in the house. I became very terrified and realized something was horribly amiss. Without another hesitation, I ran past this door streaming with hot smoke to the outside. Mr. Hive ran out too. Once outside, I was shocked to find a huge blaze of fire from the rear of the house. The roof and iron sheets where burning. The house was completely engulfed in thick black smoke and fire right up to the roof in just a short time of our escape from it. Immediately, I realized how narrowly we escaped with our lives. We did not even manage to save anything from the house. Things happened very fast; the fire was too fast and spread very quickly. I don't know what would cause a fire that starts so suddenly and spreads so fast to involve the whole house in just a short time," she explained.

At this point, several people from the Hospital and District Medical Office had made their way to the police station and were listening to her statement. Tension and great sense of loss resonated from all their faces. The scene was reminiscent of a Funeral gathering. I noticed some had tears streaming down their somber faces. One face I remember vividly was that of the Hospital Administrator; He was crying, his small eyes burnt intensely red. Looking at him, made me sense how much he was absorbing my loss.

He took in all my pain as if it was his own and I struggled hard to restrain myself from wanting to comfort him.

When the drunken officer had finished taking his statement, I asked him to take Mr. Five's story. He hesitate a while and said he could only record a statement from the legal occupant of the material house in question and not from a passerby. However, on my insistence, he reluctantly allowed Mr. Five to give his statement.

"Tell us, what did you see Five?" the Sergeant asked looking at him straight in the eye.

"I was standing in the Girl's bedroom and I saw a mattress burning,'" he started saying

"Five! What where you doing gazing into the Girl's bedroom?' came a sharp snap from the Sergeant.

"No, I didn't see anything; there was a lot of smoke...." Mr. Five retracted his own opening sentence. "Instead I was standing at the window; and I saw a child playing with matches on the mattress."

"Are you drunk sir; don't waste our time here. Just admit there is nothing you saw ..." rebuked the Sergeant, in his harsh military voice.

"Madam if you don't have any further comments, I will close your statement here. Is there anything unusual you noticed or witnessed at the house," continued the sergeant after a moment's thought.

'Three weeks ago, we had a fire from the EXSCO, Electricity Extra Supply Company, line bringing power into the house. It burnt the grass fence and many people in the neighborhood gathered to put off the fire. We reported the matter to EXSCO Technicians who were in the field at the time in our area. The technician, who climbed the pole, found loose wires had caused the spark. He rewired the line and told us we were very lack as something worse would have happened to the house. He advised the house should be checked for any loose wiring in their line to the meter and beyond. This message was communicated to the owner of the house. The other thing is; there is an illegal connection from the house to the quarter outside where Mr. Five lives," she added.

On hearing this, Mr. Five cut in; "there is no illegal connection at the house. She is not telling the truth. Even her statement is made up."

"You shut up, let the Madam continue" the sergeant rebuked Five.

"We were told by technicians who came to reconnect power at the house when we first moved in. That EXSCO was investigating the matter at the time and told us not to worry as the law would soon catch up with the perpetrators," she concluded.

"Thank you very much for your statement madam, you can *go now*," the Sergeant concluded his report after reading it out to her.

GO! This came as a shock to me. Go where? It was at this point, I realized I was homeless. I had no furniture, I had no beddings, no beds, and I had no kitchen utensils. I had no food. I had nowhere to go; Banks were closed and my VISA card and passport had burnt in the house.

I had not thought of where to take my family after giving statements at the police. Nothing had been salvaged from the inferno. All my earthly possessions had been incinerated. The cloths I had on; was all that was left of my wardrobe. On this day I wore a long sleeved plain purple shirt and black trousers. This shirt had become small over the years and couldn't be tacked in for long. It slipped out when bending or when lifting my hands over my head.

I realized immediately the impact of this disaster had just begun. Darkness, I have never known before, begun to overshadow my life. I was now at the mercy of my neighbors and my friends. I felt pain at my umbilical stump. It was as if I the umbilical cord was being sewn back to my abdomen. It is much easier to cut off the cord. It is an agonizing experience to have the umbilical cord plugged back to your abdominal wall. It is excruciating to be plunged into being a homeless dependent. I felt the tears come back to my eyes. I could accept loss of property however I could not accept to become a burden to another person. To eat, drink and take up resource meant for another person's children. To become a budget item for another family, a hard working family trying hard to make ends meet themselves. To take up space in another man's house was not among my plans and to occupy his house and probably displace his innocent children to the sitting room or kitchen. .....By now the small town of Choma was rotating towards dusk. My tribulations had just begun.

I was aware, 'it is darkest before dawn'; but my circumstances were bent on darkening dawn itself.... allegation of this magnitude could turn out very ugly indeed.

I weighed my options; I thought of asking for space at the local community hall just to shelter the night ahead. I thought of erecting a tent next to the smoldering rubble of my house. I thought of moving back in with my parents 300km away from this town. I considered checking in at a cheapest lodge in town. Moving in with my parents would at least help dampen the psychological trauma my children were suffering that very moment. And I thought of moving out of town altogether; somewhere far, far away from this tragedy. While I was pondering over my options; an old man came up to me outside the police grounds console me.

"Doc, I am deeply saddened by your tragedy. Wasn't it very recent when you had a theft at your house? Now this; I am certain someone means harm on your life," he chose his words carefully. In this town Doc, there are evil people. There are people who have sold their souls to the devil himself. I don't think they are happy of the good works you are doing in the community. Just look; you have been here only a short time, but your name is in every home. We are so proud of you however these Satanists are not. You are Father Johnston returned back to us. Did you know Dr. Johnston Doc? He was an incredibly humble surgeon and a Jesuit Priest; the community loved him deeply. I think you are his reincarnate. Now Doc, to tell you the truth; houses do not just burn like that. You could be a marked man Doc. Watch your back."

Up until then; I was treating this matter as an accident pending investigation; Thoughts of possible paranormal attack begun to infiltrate my mind after listening to this old man. As I was thinking over his counsel and caution, officials from the District Medical Office and the Hospital Management came to where I was standing.

'Doc we have arranged for you to be moved to a Lodge. You will need to rest. We can think of other things in the morning.' They said.

I looked to where my wife was standing surrounded by several women; I saw the District Medical Officer (DMO) helping her to get into her personal car. She was protesting; wanting to return to the scene. However the DMO insisted this wouldn't be a good idea. It would be too traumatic. She obliged and in the next few minutes, a convoy of cars exited the police premises. Here again, the procession was reminiscent of a Funeral.

I couldn't wait to awake my horses and join the procession at the rear. I waited till the last car had driven off the police station. I felt as though I was watching my own funeral procession. It hurt very much but was glad so many had gathered to witness my passing. "Don't the scripture say; 'A good name is better than fine perfume," I thought to myself. "If all these good people could see what God sees in my heart; I wonder how many would remain standing here with me."

I knew for a good man, many people would always want to help and mourn his passing in great numbers. I didn't consider myself a good man. I was cognizant of the fact that God saw filthy rags in my heart. Like many mortals, I possessed a wicked heart and corrupt mind. Yet he chose to send his begotten son to die for me on the cross and on that dreadful July day, he added more days to my miserable earthly life by saving me from the fire. I could have perished in that fire had it happened late at night. When the last vehicle had driven off, I awoke my horses in the car park; they galloped to join the main road, leaving a plume of dust at the police station. I raced my German stallions to join the convey heading for my temporal shelter on the out skates of town.

The sun had descended low in the sky by now, preparing to set. The western horizon was still being illuminated by its golden red rays. Gazing at this golden glow on the horizon brought memories of my burning house. I wondered what was left of it and I determined in my heart to get back to the scene as soon as my family had settled in.

At the lodge, the DMO came over to where I stood, "order anything the family wants; eat, drink and rest; we will talk in the morning."

She told the inn keeper in the words of the Good Samaritan; I recited the scripture to myself; "A Man was going down from Jerusalem to Jericho, when he fell into the hands of robbers. They stripped him of his cloths, beat him and went away leaving him half dead. A priest happened to be going down the same road, and when he saw the man, he passed by on the other side. So too, a Levite, when he came to the place and saw him, passed by on the other side; But when a Samaritan, as he travelled, came where the man was; and when he saw him, he took pity on him. He went to him and bandaged his wounds, pouring on oil and wine. Then he put the man on his own donkey, took him to an inn and took care of him. Then the next day he took out two silver coins and gave them to the innkeeper. 'Look after him,' he said, 'and when I return, I will reimburse you for any extra expense you may have." Luke 10: 30-35.

"……… Let them have anything they want. Let the children get anything. I will take care of any extra expenses when I return," she said. The bible had become alive right in front of my eyes and was being acted out word for word. I knew then, the God of Abraham, Isaac and Jacob; the God of Linda, the God of my Life, God Almighty; had not abandoned me to my miserable ways. These Good Samaritans were not there by accident.

As soon as the DMO left us and my wife and kids had gone in the family suite; I left the lodge and drove to the scene. I was surprised to find still a large gathering of sympathizers at the house. The fire had died down by now but smoke still smoldered in the house. The whole roof was burnt down complete. All the rooms but one were burnt completely down. The only standing room was baby Joshua's nursery. All the baby's things had survived the fire along with everything kept in his room; among these was my only manuscript to my first hand crafted Novel.

I stood there not believing what I was seeing; the house was completely burnt down and all my household goods incinerated inside it. While I gazed, a white lady, in her late sixties, came over to where I stood. She introduced herself as Mrs. Evans;

"I am so sorry about your tragedy," she said. "Do you have anywhere to go?"

"Everything is lost...." I tried to find words to communicate my sticky situation. "We have been lodged at Ubuntu in the out skates of town. Thank you for your concern."

"I am glad to hear that the humans have been taken care of. I see you have pets. Who is taking care of your dogs? I can take your dogs in and look after them till you are settled. And if there is anything else I can do, I will do it. Just let me know. Here is my business card," she offered. "What is the name of this big guy? He looks like a bull Mastiff."

"You are right, Major is a bull Mastiff. This here is Spike, he is a cross breed between a German Shepherd and a Rottweiler," I answered pushing Major away who was jumping all over me and hitting me with his large paws.

"The dogs seem to read your loss," Mrs. Evans observed.

"Spike is unusually cold, he is not even wagging his tail," I agreed.

"I don't have any shirts or trousers but I can give you my dress if you don't mind," she remarked as a warm humorous smile lit her English face.

I laughed with her. Her humor was exactly what I needed at that moment. I held her hand and found peace flow into my heart. She gave me a feeling like I had just met someone I had known for many years. Yet I was meeting her for the very first time. I looked at her smiling face and realized she was fighting back tears which were building up in her blue eyes; soon, they came gashing out. She sniffed hard and blew her nose. The pain of my loss was affecting her deeply and visibly. I needed to say something; something to lighten her up. The kindness she poured out to me was too generous to return mere thank you words. I needed wisdom to converse with her, however all wise words had left me. So I simply reflected on the dress she was offering me. I knew she meant more than a dress. She was willing to help my family even if it meant giving her own garments to cloth us and even offered to care for my dogs. How often does one stumble on kindness this profound. I knew immediately I just spoke with an Angel.

"I wonder how I would look like in your dress. I should go modeling in it?" I pulled her leg.

She burst out laughing when I said this. She wore a Victorian dress adorned in old English embroidery. I pictured myself in one of her old English dresses and smiled.

Later that evening, I reflected on the goodness of God even amidst great suffering. I couldn't understand the meaning of this tragedy. I couldn't even tell whether Satan had a hand in it. I found I couldn't pray. I was afraid I would just start grumbling and speak senseless words. I decided to wait on Yahweh to give me the right words to use.

As the night stretched on, it became very cold. I started thinking of the kids. They did not have any cloths to change into the following day. They did not have warm clothing. They did not have shoes. All their cloths had burnt in the house. While I thought these things, my wife spoke up;

'Honey, I have a confession to make,' she started.

My heart missed a beat. "Confess!? What is this confession all about?" I thought to myself and then I nodded for her to go ahead.

"You know last night …; I woke up to pray in the sitting room. I had a frightening experience and I decided not to tell you. A few minutes after kneeling down to pray; I felt a strong urge to ask God to pass over us; I couldn't utter any words but Lord Pass over us, Lord Pass over us. I continued repeating these words not understanding why I was saying them. Then all of a sudden, I felt a hot fiery sensation descend upon my head from the ceiling. I was so terrified that I ran to the baby's room to sleep and keep quiet about this incidence. I thought this was probably the way people that experience the Holy Spirit felt. Do you think it has anything to do with our survival from that fire?' she narrated her unusual midnight encounter.

"I have a confession too. Three days ago, I had the most bizarre nightmare. You know I have never had a nightmare before or wake up screaming in my sleep. That night in my dream; I was in our bedroom and three strange looking beings were in the room. In my dream I awoke and found these hideous looking beings had nailed three bodies on the corners of the ceiling.

One of the hideous creatures had a face of someone I know in this town and appeared to have been in charge of this legion of demons. I struggled to free myself from their grip. They wanted to nail me to the remaining slot, they had prepared for me, in the ceiling. I fought back, kicked and screamed the name of Jesus till they let go of me. Just then, I woke up. In the morning and in the last three days, I have been looking at the ceiling and roof; asking myself what death hangs over our heads in this ceiling. What sort of Death would come from the Ceiling and the Roof? I am certain; God prevented this tragedy from hitting the house at night. I don't think we would have survived it had it come at night. God gave you those utterances; Pass over us, Pass over us! ...... What he gave you was an intercessory prayer. The Angel of death had been in the house these past few days." I told her and she begun to cry terrified by the wonders of God.

I let her cry and reflect on her maker. He had just used her to save her family and strengthen her heart for the accusations ahead and forces intent on breaking the family. Had it not been for this encounter, I doubt I could have managed to comfort her from the loss of her several pairs of shoes, her washing machines, four plate cooker, her PVR decoder; her one week old Sofa, her cloths etc. She would have mourned the whole night, and probably opt to curse God like Job's Wife in the bible and vow to leave town immediately. I was very sure; she met God Almighty the night of her strange prayer. I knew she would still be targeted in the months ahead and if she faltered in her faith, Satan would do what he failed to achieve on this night. In the subsequent months, I knew the task before her would be to desist from conduct likely to open her to demonic influences and satanic mugging.

Women have been known to receive phenomenal supernatural rescue only to fall prey to the Sin of Lottie's wife in the bible; she turned into a pillar of salt and remained behind. She forgot to obey; she did not heed the LORD's command…. Don't look back…

In the meantime, I lamented my own loss: my PC and the data saved on it; the Linda manuscripts and several projects saved on the desk top, my assignments and research papers. My Reference Medical Text Books, my 32GB touch iPod; and my theater videos, the Audio Bible and the Drug reference, *epocrates* saved on it. The souvenirs, the miniature portraits of family and friends, my photo album; the list was endless; above all, the house I called my home.

Then I reflected on an amazing incidence that happened in the family two weeks previously. My wife had wanted to name our one week old son. I rejected all the names she presented to me. She eventually got angry and gave up.

"You go ahead and name him yourself," she had snapped at me angrily.

"His name will be Matauka, after your uncle in Lusaka. He is the first person I knew in your family," I proposed.

"NO! all boys given that name in my family do not live to survive childhood. He can't be called Matauka," She refused vehemently.

"If that name carries death; I refuse Death to come into my house. His name shall be called Joshua; because Joshua means; 'God Saves'," I pronounced him firmly.

"But... Joshua! Why Joshua? I know God saves but what are we being saved from this time?" she protested.

"I don't know what he is saving us from however his name is Joshua and that's final," I answered and walked out of the house.

Meanwhile in our Hotel room, the clock struck midnight. I proposed we try to catch some sleep. Baby Joshua was sleeping by her side. I gazed at the baby as he slept peacefully.

"Joshua!" the mention of his name evoked a sense of awe. God had given me his name two weeks prior to the burning of the house. "What sort of a baby is this one that is named of God?" I thought to myself.

At the Burning House, his room and his things survived the inferno. Was this a coincidence? I was sure it couldn't be. I was convinced God had saved my family. And with that, I allowed sleep to envelop my eyes. It had been a long stressful day.

I was woken up by loud voices outside. It was morning and the sun had ascended the skies already taking command of the day. I didn't realize I had been so tired. I slept right through the night. A sizeable gathering was outside to greet us. I recognized a pastor clutching a Bible. I realized, these must be people from one congregation in town.

The pastor led us through the morning devotions and blessed the day ahead. Then one man gave a testimony which was told to him by a patient of mine at Macha Girls High School. We were greatly encouraged by it. He narrated how a Teacher of Mathematics woke up his wife in the early hours of the morning; the same day our house burnt. He was an Elder at a local church and someone I knew. His wife was a God fearing woman. She was a person I greatly respected in their church.

He narrated quoting the words of the school teacher…"around 03 hours yesterday, I received a strong conviction that there was going to be a tragedy somewhere to someone we knew," he said. "I immediately woke up my wife so that we could pray….. *"Bana Musenge bukeni tupepe"*; *(Honey wake up we pray)* I said; but she was too tired to join me. So I prayed alone till morning. When she woke up at day break, she told me, while I prayed; she had a dream in which she saw a house burning. Then she remarked firmly, honey; today, there will be a house that will burn somewhere; belonging to someone we know very well. I reassured her that God had shown me there would be no loss of life. And so when we heard our doctor's house had burnt down, we were very terrified but we praised God, him alone knows why the house had to burn."

Shortly after they left, a young beautiful Nigerian Doctor, Dr Nkechi Ounowchi, came over to see us. She was a volunteer at the Hospital where I worked. She was crying and visibly shaken by our calamity. She was the most unlikely person to express the emotions she was displaying in our hotel room. Those that knew Dr Nkechi, will tell you, her outward appearances told of a girl that loved the fast life, and lived a somewhat care free life, she appeared to have no time for empathy or any attachment to those going through pain and suffering. She dressed like a Model; often preferring quite revealing skirts. In this conservative community, few understood her. It took me until that day to understand her and see an Angel hidden inside her heart; and made me vow never again to Judge a person by the cloths they wore.

"I am so sorry about your loss; and the children, this must be very traumatic for them," she spoke with her beautiful Nigerian Accent. "I am only remaining with three months in your country. I want you to move into my house. I'll move out to a lodge or a guest house. This way; the children can have a sense of a home again. The shorter this transition takes the better for them. They shouldn't be let to sense this horrifying loss. I think this will help heal the traumatic scenes they witnessed yesterday… before it is registered in their subconscious mind. My house is fully furnished and is self-contained and has a working geyser. There is cable TV, they can watch cartoons. I have enough food in the house to last several weeks; you can have it," She spoke firmly and wept incessantly with a sincere Nigerian etiquette to display loss.

"This can't be happening; I must be watching a Nigerian Movie. She must be out of her Mind," I thought to myself.

I tried protesting and refused to inconvenience her. This Accommodation was meant to make her two years stay in Zambia comfortable and a memorable one. It was located in the prime area of Choma in Mochipapa road. It was part of her Government's incentive of looking after its Citizens away from home.

My protests didn't work. She rushed to her house and picked her cloths and moved out to a Lodge. This is how my family moved into a fully furnished house and those who came to see us in subsequent days could not believe a fire had burnt our house.

We appeared to have everything overnight. The kids were watching their favorite cartoons and running around the house in Tom and Jerry pursuits. For them it was business as usual.

My son even remarked, "Dad; how come you that woman gave you a house. You have got back all your things in just one day. How come? As for me; my bicycle has not come back to me yet."

It was Jay that made this observation. As far as the kids were concerned, it was now a competition to see who got most of their things back.

Dr. Nkechi's sacrifice healed an entire family. I called her selfless acts; 'The Nigerian Prescription." I still thank her deeply to this very day. I don't think *'THANK'* is the correct word. I must say; I still *REVERE* her actions to this very day. She taught me never to judge a woman by the cloths she chooses to wear in this life.

I think fashion and dress are an Enigma to those blinded by prejudice in this Fashion Conscious Age. A woman should be judged by the contents of her heart and not by the length of her skirt.

In the following days; the course of God's River of life flowed through our newly acquired home, bringing along amazing people I could never have dreamt lived among us. Ordinary people, among them my patients trekked to our home and blessed us in diverse ways. The white farmers of Choma sent us numerous gifts. Ordinary people of Choma swarmed our new home with all sort of gifts; blankets, mattresses, pots, plates, food, clothing etc.; one man from 'Sale Na Sale' brought my children a Television set and DVD player; then a cheerful Lady, I later learnt to be Mrs. Scott, drove to our house and brought us sofas;

"God has placed this need on my heart to give you these lovely seats, I hope you like them," she said and drove off as quickly as she had come.

Gifts kept coming visitor after visitor; each instructed by God on a specific need area. There was never duplication of the things each one brought us. A clear sign this wasn't some random or haphazard order of events. The Hand of God was guiding and healing us every step of the way.

Seeing this, I decided we would not ask for anything from anyone. I realized God knew our specific needs. He had already decided what we should have. And so when people asking me to write a list of things I wanted them to buy for us called on us; I firmly told them I could not do such a thing.

I told one entourage that came to my house, "I am afraid to say what I want. I do not know what God wants me to have. He has taken everything away but has preserved my life and that of my family; I cannot ask anything beyond this. If I say I want shoes or I want that; I might sin against him. I do not have the wisdom to ask what he wants me to have. I do not know what he is teaching me through this. I don't understand anything or what is coming in the months ahead. Therefore I can't ask for anything. Not because I have anything but because I do not have the wisdom to ask him to tell me what I must ask from you. I do not know what he wants me to have."

And if you are among these amazing people living among us that came to my home or stayed in your secrete chambers of your home and prayed for my family or simply sent your gift through a friend or other, I have this to say;

I thank God for having used you to easy my suffering. I wish I could write your name on the pages of this book. But I won't; instead I will engrave your name on the walls and Chambers of my HEART; the Temple of the Holy Spirit who guided your prayers and Love gifts to my family. In this way; I hope to bring your name to have an everlasting dwelling in the presence of God Almighty. I pray that your gift offering may be returned to you a 100fold. However that would be too little, allow me then to say; may my God repay your kindness and may it be given back to you abundantly and 'without measure.'

As with any human event, good or bad; Time rolled on; Days stretched into weeks; weeks gave way to months; the cold season was succeeded by the hot season. The Presidential and parliamentary election came and the MMD government was thrown out and in its place came the Patriotic Front Government. The face of the losing president was pulled down from office walls and the face of Mr. Sata now greeted you in public offices and private business offices. I gazed at his face, during a visit to a public office, and drew lots of inspiration from his resilience....; at 70, he was still looking youthful and strong to soldier on.... It was a long walk to state house... "Long walk to Plot One" great title for his book... should he consider one, I thought to myself. The losing candidate had it easy.... He inherited the presidency. I dreaded, the day a scoundrel would steal the presidency in our beautiful country. I was aware evil lurked around in dark corners seeking corruptible men and women to ensnare.

Anyhow...that's the order of the passing of time; then the rain season came and watered the land. But the memory of my calamity refused to fade away from my mind. Darkness hovered on and the breeze of a good morning tarried on. With the coming of the rains, I wished my house had been savannah grassland because then new healthier grass and shrubs would have sprouted where the old dry grass had burnt. On the contrary, these were brick walls and cement floors; the rains only added to the grotesque site of a desolate place. Shrubs and all manner of plants of the wild, including vegetables, grew in the living room where my children once played happily.

I stood in this uninhabited living room, during one visit to my scorched house, and saw how 'life after people' laid claim to my deserted dwellings. The house was metamorphosing into a dwelling place for the kingdom Animalia and the plant kingdom. As I looked, a Hairy Black Spider from the family Pholcidea emerged from a crack in the wall to stalk a Bee from the family Apidae. In the corner, I noticed the spider spanned a web; a perfect trap requiring only a wrong flight bearing by the worker Bee and she would be dinner for the Spider Pholcidea family.

"This is Kingdom Animalia my friend, you have to watch your back," I thought to myself as I strode out of the house.

Gossip was ripe in the community on the burning of the house; you couldn't blame people take sides; while I was celebrating the goodness of God; Evil men lurked all over town and were determined to find my family guilty of burning the house. A community such us ours was never short of scoundrels and rumor-mongers. Even so, I won't waste your time to write about their spiteful slander and malice. However, all I want you to know is this, "Blessed is the man that walketh not in the counsel of the ungodly, nor standeth in the way of sinners, nor siteth in the seat of the scornful. But his delight is in the Law of the Lord; and in his Law doth he meditate day and night. And he shall be like a tree planted by the rivers of water, that bringeth forth his fruit in his season; his leaf also shall not wither; and whatsoever he doeth shall prosper.

Some officers from the local police station exercised exemplary professionalism in handling the case of my burnt house. While evil men were scheming to cast the blame on my family; God was watching over us and prevented corrupt police officers from casting the blame on us.

The reports from other officials charged with investigating the cause of the fire were like a child's writing. Total lack of professionalism characterized handling and reporting the evidence gathered or lack of it. The Electricity Company, EXSCO, on one hand refused to furnish the investigating officer with a technical report saying a rumor-monger had told them fire started on a mattress, and so they stated through their crooked company lawyer, they couldn't be involved with the investigation. I couldn't understand how a power company could sink so low as to listen to rumor on a matter as serious as this?

This lack of professionalism from some sectors, especially EXSCO and the Combustion Company would lead to the climax of the events which begun on a bright July afternoon. A court hearing which I won before the matter even started. Mr. Five chose to sue me on behalf of his family seeking compensation from me and submitted that I build him a new house when he could have sued the electricity company. Every sane person knew of course, the power company was responsible for the fire that burnt my house.

It had been nine long months of; rumor, bigotry, prejudice, uncertainty, and extreme emotional trauma for me and my family before the matter went to court. I tried to concentrate at work, however I found this was wearying me down. I decided to take a vacation leave without any intention of ever returning to this community I had come to love. I knew I would miss all my friends and the good people I met, especially my patients. However, I knew I couldn't stay; something worse than fire itself happened and strengthened my resolve to leave; I was already anxiously looking forward to my new station and the work awaiting me and the struggle of starting a new life when the ugly cold hand of betrayal came lurking into my house; the one house fire failed to burn down. But betrayal laid it bare and inhospitable. Anyhow, that's a very long story. I know the flames of gossip and rumor will spread it…… I must remain strong and stay focused; the way to eternal life is long and tortuous; I must leave some people here while I go yonder to pray…God Saves.

And so it was; one late evening, on a Sunday, while I was thinking over the hideous nature of betrayal and unfaithfulness; I was not surprised to receive a summon requiring me to present myself at the Laws and Regulations Foundation without fail. My landlord made a move I had been waiting for all nine months. He had sort legal recourse in the matter.

What followed was an epic battle at dawn; it was about to turn very dark in my life. I wished I had lingered long enough during a visit to my desolate house to see what happened between the Pholcidea and the Apidae families…… but I knew the bright rays of morning were coming; so I waited;

During this trying time, I drew great lessons from the life of an incredible young Lady who was nursing someone very close to her while at the same time preparing to take her final Year University Examinations. Her faith in God profoundly touched my heart and inspired a friendship that unleashed my own healing. 'Sunset at Noon' is a memoir to this Friendship. Her mother was my patient, and as the events at this point in my life unfolded…. Her mother was taken critically ill….; I had booked her for urgent surgery to check what it was that was obstructing her intestines; but the 'cold hand of betrayal' prevented me at the last hour…. And so I hastily made a call to my reliable surgical friend to take over the patient…. I was very sad to see my friend and my patient leave. The events that would follow rendered my lamentations trivial. This young lady would shoulder the heaviest load known to man. It made me laugh at my predicaments.

In the mean time I considered talking to a lawyer what to expect at such Hearings. Instead I decided the God that saved my family would not abandon me at such a critical hour.

My labor pains were swift and unrelenting; ready to birth in a new life. The hearing was a spectacle like none I have attended before. Emotions and Tampers ran high to echo the high temperatures pounding the city of Livingstone. In the distance, the mighty Victoria Falls roared and thundered to the amusement of the visiting tourists. I was a free man determined to start all over again and make Livingstone my new home.

The Promise

The ordeal that left her with an indelible Scar broke my spirit and cut her heart too deep to mend. I reflected at how many women suffered such avoidable injuries in a civilized society. I bemoaned the state of poor maternity care in rural areas; a notoriety that was an indictment of the wild third world in the 21st Century.

It was the worst birth injury I have seen in years. I couldn't imagine how she managed to walk. The pain she was under was beyond description. I could almost feel it on myself, emanating from the chair I sat on. Notwithstanding being a man; and though my knowledge of Human Anatomy was remarkable, I stared at the injury in total bewilderment.

I had thoroughly studied the anatomy of the female man region by region; however, looking at the patient before me that morning made me look like a novice on the subject. I couldn't identify basic landmarks. I couldn't point out the opening for urine, the passage for stool and the birth canal. There was simply one opening for urine, stool and for birthing. The walls that form a boundary to this sensitive and private territory were all heavily swollen and engorged with fluid and hang several centimeters from their rightful position in the normal; both urine and stool were exiting her body via the birth canal. Urine was dripping continuously as she had lost control of voiding it willfully. Her left leg was paralyzed and she used a walking stick to steady herself and supplement the weakness in her leg. A distressing malodorous whiff of Urine attended her company like a demon rapt on tormenting her.

Her ordeal started the day she went into labor; seeing that labor had started suddenly at 9pm, before the expected date of confinement, she rushed to the local clinic where she was admitted immediately. She was kept for two days at the rural clinic and was told her labor was too slow. By the second day, she was told labor had entered the active phase and was moved into labor ward to await delivery. And so she waited and waited till night fall but her baby did not come. By now she was extremely exhausted and sleep deprived. The health worker that checked her birthing passage reported it to be 7cm earlier that day and was still 7 cm the following day. At this point, the clinic decided to refer the patient to the nearest district hospital, some two hours away on public transport, with a carefully written out referral; it read:

"We refer the patient for further management due to prolonged progress of labor and fetal Distress."

Sadly, her baby would not make it to the district hospital. It died in the womb half an hour shy of the hospital. This was confirmed by ultra sound scanning at the District Hospital. She was too tired to mourn the loss of her first born baby. She had cried her last tear, mourning the anguish of labor she had been through and now, she just wanted to be set free from this persecution and fall asleep. She was in GSD, Great Sleep Deprivation.

The effect of sleep deprivation on a woman in labor rarely gets the attention it deserves or is not understood at all. Often the patient is blamed for being uncooperative and when she loses her baby, trying to deliver, is reported as; 'the baby died due to poor maternal effort.' How can anyone expect a sleep deprived woman to cooperate and follow instructions? Great sleep deprivation mimics psychosis and drunkenness. It leads to distorted perception, inappropriate emotional and behavioral responses. Twenty one hours of sleep deprivation is equivalent to a blood alcohol content of 0.8% which is the blood alcohol limit for drunk driving in the United States of America, Great Britain and Canada. The legal limit in most Western Nations is 0.5%.

It has long been known that sleepy driving is as bad as drunken driving; if not worse. Let it be known to all who read this that 'Sleep Deprived moms' in Labor are in far worse mental state than drunken drivers on our roads.

The point is; a woman should never be allowed to labor when she is found to be at high risk for sleep deprivation.. Or put simply; never let the Sun Set on a woman in Labor.

It is immoral to shout at a sleep deprived patient in labor. It must be remembered that sleep deprivation causes the brain to become incapable of putting an emotional event into the proper perspective and is incapable of making a controlled suitable response to the event.

Health workers looking after mothers in labor should always aim at identifying these mothers and expedite their birthing. It is no wonder many relatives try to expedite labor using herbal Oxytocic concoctions and often with disastrous consequences.

A woman should not be allowed to enter a phase of micro sleeps during the second stage of labor. Micro sleeps occur when a person has a significant sleep deprivation. The brain automatically shuts down, falling into a sleep state for a period that can last from a second to half a minute. The person falls asleep no matter what activity he or she is engaged in.

Micro sleeps are similar to blackouts and a person experiencing them is not consciously aware that they are occurring. It is not surprising to find a woman falling asleep when it is time to push her baby out; a period known as the second stage of labor.

Many women lose babies in this stage of labor and are unfairly blamed by the attending health worker for poor maternal effort; And sometimes by their spouses and families for being lazy. For goodness sake, the woman was too tired to even cooperate. Her womb was too tired to. And sometimes a woman might even die because her womb was too tired to contract resulting into excessive bleeding; a condition referred to as Atonic Uterus.

To understand how dangerous sleep deprivation is; try getting on a Bus with a drunken driver at the wheel from Nakonde to Livingstone. The point is; a woman in labor should never be left to suffer sleep deprivation let alone a complicated delivery.

Unfortunately for my patient, more anguish awaited her at the district hospital. It was decided, since the baby had died, she be delivered via the birth canal. It turned out to have been a very big baby, weighing 4.5kg. And owing to the baby's big size, in a first time mom of small stature.... Her Delivery would be awfully gruesome to pen down. Her groaning, moans, shouts, howls, yells, screams, shrieks, hollers and cries for help could be heard for miles away.

Since returning from my post graduate studies, that I cut short, in the prestigious school of medicine –Directorate of postgraduate studies, I set up office in maternity wanting to be closest to my patients.

I met Chanda on one of my usual busy days at my rural office in Chief Macha's chiefdom. She narrated her ordeal, with torrents of tears streaming down her face in my consultation room. I was left speechless.

This was not my first case of birth injury to attend. However, each human emotion is unique and always my first.

Chanda was a professional woman working for the civil service and stationed in one of the rural communities of the country. She worked on the northern part, close to the border between Zambia and Malawi. She had heard about our humble mission hospital and crossed many towns and hospitals to seek a consultation with us.

I concluded my examination and decided this injury was extremely extensive for my skills to handle.

"I am so sorry Chanda, you had to travel this far…," I began to speak.

"Doc, distance is not a problem. All I want is to get well," she said wiping tears from her eyes.

"Personally, I have not repaired an injury this big; I only have theoretical knowledge on how to repair your injury and I wouldn't want to make you my first patient. However, I know someone who can repair it. He is my teacher and taught me what I know today. He is usually very busy and difficulty to find. I will call him just now and tell him about you. Please do not go to any one else just because they repair things. This injury requires special skills which I do not yet possess. Only a few doctors have these skills and my teacher is among the few I know," I spoke plainly and was astonished by my own sincerity.

Chanda remained quiet. Absorbing every word I spoke. She listened to my telephone conversation and was delighted to know my Teacher would be pleased to see her immediately.

"I am so sorry again, I couldn't help you Chanda," I said when I had put my Nokia eleven hundred away.

"But you just did Doc, you found me someone to see and you have even booked an appointment for me. You have been the most sincere doctor I have ever met. Thank you very much," Chanda explained cheering up.

She reached out in her purse and pulled several notes to pay me. I carefully held her hand and reminded her about the journey ahead;

"The journey ahead is still very long honey. You will need every kwacha you have on you. Please accept when I say you must hold on to this money," I carefully worded my refusal to be paid.

"Thank you so much Doc; you have greatly lightened my load. I feel as though I have been healed already. I can no longer feel the pain and anguish that have tormented me this past month. Sorrow has been my constant companion and sleep has been far from my eyes. Irrepressible tears have wet my pillow night after night. I think, for the first time in many weeks; I will sleep tonight. You have taken my sorrow away just like that. My trip was indeed worthwhile. God should send many Doctors like you," Chanda spoke choosing her words like a Psalmist.

I extended my hand to say goodbye, however she chose to embrace me and hugged me good bye. I held her hand, after the passionate hug she gave me, and instead of saying goodbye; I found myself making her a promise.

"Honey, next time you are expecting, please let me know. I do not want you to go through the ordeal of labor ever again. I will deliver your baby by caesarean section. I want you to deliver at the hospital where I shall be. As long as I am alive, I want you to have a safe delivery; both you and your baby," I spoke with sincerity in my heart.

"I don't know what to say; I don't know how to thank you doc..." Chanda started to say with tears running down her face and her voice muffled by the overwhelming emotions unleashed in her heart by *the promise.*

Chanda was a high spirited girl and extremely out going. Unfortunately, this tempest had persecuted her beyond her limit and she was beginning to break down. Our meeting seemed to have rejuvenated her sunken zeal for life and put a smile on her face. This was evident in her phone call the following day.

"Hi my good Doctor; how are you today? I met your Teacher and he was so good that he made me forget I was a patient. He has given me an appointment; he says I see him in three months to allow for the swelling to go down and the body to start attempts at healing itself first. He told me if he tried to operate on me now, the Fistulae would not heal. This kind of edema, as he put it, is not good for wound healing; let alone fistulae repair…," Chanda lectured me on Fistula Surgery.

"I am delighted for you. Where are you going to be these three months, while waiting for the appointment?" I asked and avoided commenting on the lecture about Fistula Surgery she had just delivered to me.

She returned to her province extremely satisfied and happy. Week after week, Chanda called to greet me and report on her healing progress.

It was only a month later that I applied my mind to settle Chanda's case in my mind. A lot had gone wrong since the day of her admission at the rural clinic.

Being a first time mother and carrying a big baby, the clinic should have referred her immediately to the district hospital. It was unacceptable the clinic kept her that long.

All antenatal mothers carrying High Risk Pregnancies ought to be referred immediately. In Obstetrics we say; patients who come to hospital with extensive birth injuries such as Chanda's, are 'the survivors'. Most mothers die following excessive hemorrhage ensuing from such injuries.

The day I attended Chanda, I was struck by deep awe attending a survivor of the perils of child birth lurking in rural areas. Perils shared by many women in third world countries. Perils that so many girls; the future mothers, know nothing about.

I hope by the discourse of this writing, I may make known these vexations and call to conference their remedy. And so it was; day after day, week after week; I thought about Chanda; I then turned my mind to reflect on the lecture she had given me over the phone after the Fistula Surgeon had attended her and given her an appointment;

In medicine, a Fistula is an abnormal connection or passage between two epithelium lined organs or vessels that normally do not connect. It is generally a disease condition however a fistula may be surgically created for therapeutic reasons.

In obstetrics, fistula is a severe medical condition in which a hole or communication develops between either; the rectum and the vagina or between the urinary bladder and the vagina. These are referred to as Rectovaginal Fistula and Vesicovaginal Fistula respectively. They result after severe or failed childbirth, when adequate medical care is not available.

The fistula usually develops when a prolonged labor presses the unborn baby so tightly in the birth canal that blood flow is cut off to the surrounding tissues, which necrotize and eventually rot away. More rarely, the injury can be caused by poorly performed abortions, or a pelvic fracture. Other potential direct causes for fistula are sexual abuse and rape. Risk factors include; early pregnancies in teen girls, having a big baby, small stature mom, lack of access to emergency obstetric care etc.

Symptoms and signs of fistula are; urine or fecal incontinence, which maybe continually or happen at night.

The resulting disorders typically include severe infections and ulcerations of the vaginal tract, and often paralysis caused by nerve damage. Sufferers from this disorder are usually subject to severe social stigma due to odor, perception of uncleanness, a mistaken assumption of sexually transmitted infections and, in some cases, the inability to have children.

"How true of Chanda's ordeal and many forgotten women in several rural areas around Africa," I thought to myself.

While I was wrestling memories about Chanda's ordeal; I met a young couple who narrated an ordeal so vexing that I made them Chanda's Promise. Two years previously; they had waited the birth of their daughter with great longing, as do most newlyweds. They had chosen the hospital to have their baby so carefully that nothing was left to chance. Nothing could be anticipated to go wrong. The reputation of their choice hospital far exceeded any in the region.

The nine months waiting were soon reduced to labor ward hours...hours shared intricately by anxious waiting relatives and the laboring mother. Unknown to the couple, the chief of obstetrics was away from the hospital on this day; in attendance where his students... These were Medical licentiates and Interns that had recently graduated from Medical School.

The alert Midwives had noted this labor to be abnormal however the young doctors refused to take instruction from the Midwives. They thought themselves too senior to listen to midwives.

They neglected the simple rule of maternity care; 'Caring for a pregnant woman is never a contest for Heroism or a Battle of wits. It is a virtuous call of Duty to help the woman birth her child safely and healthy.'

Seeing the attendants to be unrepentant in their pride and resolve, the midwives recoiled in submission to their new lieutenants. And penitently took orders to observe the patient another six hours. The result was catastrophic. The patient had already labored beyond acceptable limit and the six hours extension, by these novices, would be a death sentence for the young infant.

The baby was born severely Asphyxiated; this is to say, the baby could not move or cry as expected of new born babies. It had been deprived of oxygen and its brain cells irreversibly damaged. The young mother watched helpless as frantic efforts were being made to revive her new born baby. The relatives waited anxiously to hear the cry of the new born baby… however none came.

The couple would spend the next year traversing 600km from their rural post to Lusaka for follow up in the pediatric neurology clinic. The Diagnosis was heart breaking; Cerebral Palsy of the worst degree. This was the most tormenting period in the life of this young couple. Intense Grief never left the presence of their new home. No words of mouth could comfort them in their anguish. And within a year of untold misery and grief, their baby would be returned to heaven; causing them to stomach yet another heart breaking memory in their young life; one that advances interrogations whose answers berg to question the very meaning of life itself. We met three years after I met Chanda and I was privileged to share in their happiness the following year.

Having left Chief Macha's chiefdom, my meandering road would take me to the small district hospital of in the country; here I quickly put my Obstetric skills in service to the mothers of this small town. The midwives of this district hospital were the best I have worked with during my sojourn and in my ever drifting road ahead.

Having watched me carefully, discharging my duties diligently, this young couple asked me to attend the delivery of their baby. They narrated their chilling ordeal in their previous pregnancy and pleaded with me to attend their delivery. I was greatly humbled by their trust.

And truly by the next year, the wife was heavy with child; I was privileged to attend her antenatal. A cheerful young lady she was and diligent in her work. She was a registered nurse at the same district hospital I worked and her husband an enthusiastic local school teacher. So great was the trust I received from them that it was beginning to make me nervous. However, I was comforted by the constant thought that this was God's work and not my own. So I simply placed everything in his hands and waited for the set dates.

Meanwhile 1000 km away to the north of our district hospital, Chanda was heavy with child too. Time had passed so fast and the promise was now only weeks away. She made arrangements to make the long journey to see me. It was a delightful meeting notwithstanding in a few days, I would inflict a wound on her abdomen to deliver her baby. I couldn't believe, it had been four years since we last met in my rural office.

The malodorous urine demon that tormented her life had left her. I figured it had been successfully exorcised by the Fistula Surgeon I sent her to see. I couldn't bring myself to ask how her operation was. This was not a good time to resurrect the past. The work ahead required great veneration. An Elective caesarean section can be a perilous undertaking as I found out once with a patient I called Sandra.

Chanda had travelled over 900km seeking the promise I made her four years earlier. Four years was such a long time to keep a life and death promise... but there she was beaming with joy and trusting my surgical skills were still sharp; and not rusted or perhaps gone blunt by months of disuse . She made it seem the promise was made just the other day.

I decided to fulfill the promise I made to the young couple and delayed Chanda's by a week. This was to allow her settle down from her long journey and to acclimatize.

The day of surgery came; the young couple entered theatre like a pair of Siamese twins joined to the hospital trolley; the wife on the trolley and the husband by her side. I had determined to conduct the operation under spinal anesthesia; this is to say, to knock out sensation from the patient's waist downwards. This would keep the patient awake throughout the operation and enable her to see her baby when it was born.

As for her loving husband, I planned to have him cut the umbilical cord. This is not a standard of care to be copied by my readers. I had, at this point in my practice, perfected my skill for caesarean section to mastery level and surrendered these skills to the glory of God. I determined to conduct a C section as though it were a normal delivery. My patients were fed a full diet soon after the surgery and placed on oral medications and generous pain killers. My patients were encouraged to walk within eight hours of surgery to reduce the risk of blood clotting in the large veins of their legs. I ensured never to touch a patient's intestines during surgery. This way, the intestines never became sluggish in their movements as seen when surgeons waste time touching them.

I had also devised a 'Commando' Operation to storm the abdomen and womb so fast that the body wouldn't even realize I had freed the baby held hostage inside the mother's womb. In this way, the armies of the body, referred to as the immune system, would not be angered to mobilize a counter attack on the wounds I would create and leave behind.

The Generals and body Marshals would be too busy celebrating the joy of the mother and her baby suckling at the breast to send destroyer bombers to the wound let alone halt the movements of her intestines.

The only direction the soldiers of her immune system could flow would be towards the breast and out through the milk into the newborn. Here, their role is to Aid the young earthling combat germs in the environment, on this perilous planet, for the next several months.

And so it was, with great skill and by the grace of God, I delivered the baby and the theatre nurse handed the scissors to the husband to cut the baby's cord. He cut it overwhelmed by paternity love and not too sure his baby would feel the pain. There was great jubilation in theatre. I held the baby and lifted it for the mother to see. She was so overjoyed that tears rolled freely down her cheeks. Her husband, who had come round the operating table, kissed his wife, as they shared their mutual gratitude to God; their offspring was born without any complications.

The following week came and I entered theatre once again to perform this delicate ceremony; the birth of a baby by caesarean section.

Chanda lay on the operating table not scared at all or troubled about anything. She trusted me completely…;

I longed for this kind of trust; 'If I could have it, I would express it to my God in heaven,' I thought to myself.

The operation proceeded without incidence and delivered a healthy baby girl. Chanda was so overjoyed that she begged to be allowed to hold her baby whilst still on the operating table. The midwife obliged to her request and handed her the baby. It was a sight like non I have seen.

While mother and baby where making acquaintances, I busied myself to close Chanda's abdominal wound. By the time the midwife recovered the baby from its mother's loving arms, I made leave of the operating table in reverence of God. The operation had gone very well.

I was released from the Promise that bound me for four years to a stranger I met at my rural hospital. The stranger who became my friend; I felt a free man again. I was merry knowing though a man of flesh and blood, I had lived to keep a promise I made to another human being; the Promise that mended a broken heart and healed an indelible scar.

In the next six years, I went on to attend the birth of Chanda's other two beautiful babies. All were born by caesarean section at Livingston Hospital where I now worked.

***

And God shall wipe away all their tears from their eyes; and there shall be no more death, neither sorrow, nor crying, neither shall there be any more pain: for the former things are passed away. And he that sat upon the throne said, Behold, I make all things new. And he said unto me, write: for these words are true and faithful. And he said unto me, it is done. I am Alpha and Omega, the beginning and the end. I will give unto him that is thirst of the fountain of the water of life freely. He that overcometh shall inherent all things; and I will be his God and he shall be my son.

(Rev 21: 4-7)

Chasing Trails of Enlightenment

The Boeing 737 descended down towards Qingdao coastal Airport. My colleagues and I were on a guided tour of the Famous Sailing city in the North east of China.

Earlier that day, we left Baiyun international Airport aboard a Hainan Airlines and flew over three hours to Qingdao. I was part of a seventeen member team of International Medical Officials from Africa. Those who would create an indelible impression on my mind were; Dr Abel Selassie whom everyone called the Emperor, Dr William Fisher, Dr Anna Husain, James and Adams. Dr Gytano Odinga, a very difficult fellow to get along with, Dr Hercules the wrestler, Dr Georgina, an incredibly overweight hard to please doctor. Esther, who mourned daily about her African food; Dr Marximillian, a very interesting fellow and Linda the Saint; others included, Dr Mike Chomba who never got along with Gytano, Dr Rolex, Dr Oscar Uhuru, Charlie and Dr Bob Junior the politician.

The flight path took us through some spectacular landscapes seen from the sky above. The plane cruised over the clouds and sometimes, descended below them whenever the pilot had a site to show off. We crossed spectacular mountain ranges and saw China's famous Yangtze River. The pilot turned his large plane to a 15 degree angle on either side to allow his passengers to catch a glimpse of the beautiful river below.

The river ran a zig zag course through a series of mountain ranges. It meandered like a giant snake. From the aircraft above, I could see human habitations in various areas along the river. I saw a large city in one area that had sprung up along the course of the river. Several vessels could be seen from the air sailing on the Yangtze. For millennia, this river has taken this lonely course to the Pacific Ocean. Further, the Huang He River too, took a tortuous course to China's yellow sea.

When the pilot was satisfied passengers had seen enough of the river, he pointed the nose of his plane up and begun to climb. Soon we were flying far above the clouds in the sky. There were occasional windows between the clouds to look at the beautiful blue earth below.

Linda sat at the back with Dr Rolex and Charlie, both medical officials from southern Africa. In front of them, an Ethiopian medical official sat with two beautiful Chinese girls; Emma and Serena that had accompanied the team to Shandong province. On the immediate right to where Linda sat, Esther from east Africa sat with Georgina and an official from Ethiopia. The other officials from east and southern Africa sat at the front with Chinese travelers.

"Did you know, statistically we are safer here at the back than those that are seated at the front?" said Junior looking at Linda.

Linda nodded and turned to admire the clouds through her window. The clouds reminded her of Candy wrapped on long sticks she ate when she was little. She was trying to avoid getting into a discussion about fatal aircraft accidents and disappearances in recent times.

"This aircraft is amphibious; if we crashed into the sea, it can float," said Oscar.

"No! No! No; that is very difficult landing. It has only been successfully done once," I argued.

"Yes, an old pilot saved his passengers by landing his plane into the Hudson River in America," said Junior.

Marx sat quietly, his ears plugged with ear phones, in a seat two rolls in front of the beautiful Chinese girls accompanying us on a tour of Qingdao city. I sat in front of Dr Marximillian who wished he could swap a seat with the Ethiopian official seated next to Serena. Marx was upset the surgeon from Ethiopia chose to sleep leaving the beautiful girls lonely. Serena and Emma resorted to watching movies on the Tablets provided by the airline. The gods had generously given the East African official three long hours to charm the Chinese girls but he simply wasted it. Marx was angry with the airline. He thought, it should have given him the courtesy of choosing his seat mates. I was comfortable in my seat.

The Boeing 737, Hainan Airline touched down at the magnificent Qingdao international Airport at 1pm. We were received by the most gorgeous tour guide sent straight from heaven.

"My name is Snow, I will be your tour guide over the next three days of your stay here in Qingdao," she introduced herself once we were on the bus from the airport.

Snow spoke very good English with a beautiful American accent. Qingdao was her home town and she promised to make everyday memorable for the visitors. Everyone loved her immediately.

"First, I will take you for Lunch and then we will visit the famous Tsingtao beer Museum after lunch," she explained.

"Will there be beer?" Dr Abel Selassie asked.

"Yes, you will have plenty of free beer there," Snow answered smiling.

"Let's go straight for the Beer Joint then; food can wait," Oscar remarked. We all burst out laughing.

The restaurant Snow chose served a buffet of sea food; the meal we ate here was the most gorgeous food we had ever tasted since coming to china. Origus was located along Jingkou road, not far from the intersection with Fengshan road.

"This is Origus Restaurant; I hope you will find the food yummy," said Snow leading us into the spacious restaurant.

"The aroma is scrumptious. I love this restaurant already," I remarked finding a seat.

"I don't want to sit with someone asking me the nomenclature of my food," said Dr Marx taking a seat on the table where Dr Rolex and Mike sat.

The food was so delicious that Esther and Georgina found it irresistible to indulge themselves in sea food. For a moment since coming to China,

Esther forgot her Matoke while Dr Abel forgot his Injera. I served myself a large plate of Lobster and Hairy crabs. A Chinese chef passed through the tables calling 'Pizza'; he wanted us to taste the pizza he had made.

"Pizza, Pizza ...," he shouted looking left and right through the tables.

Georgina, Anna, Linda, Dr James and I where the first to heed his pizza call; as it turned out; it was the most tasty pizza I had eaten since coming to China. It was made in traditional Sino-Italiano style.

"I'll be damned if this pizza was a copy, it is truly good. Original Italian style," Georgina remarked gorging herself on a fourth piece.

Mike and Dr Rolex stuffed themselves on Shell and Oysters which they washed down with blackberry wine.

"Pizza, Pizza, Pizza," Dr Rolex called out. He was imitating the Chinese chef as he walked to help himself on pizza and fruits. Everyone burst out laughing.

When everyone had their fill, it was time to check out the beer museum.

After a fifteen minute drive from Origus, we arrived at No.56 Dengzhou, the Beer Museum. The road to the museum was lined by several restaurants specializing in beer. Everywhere my colleagues and I looked, we were greeted with the words; 'welcome to the home of beer'. Everyone, except Linda, Dr Rolex and I was gripped by thirst that transcended that for water. They could not have been happier when the bus

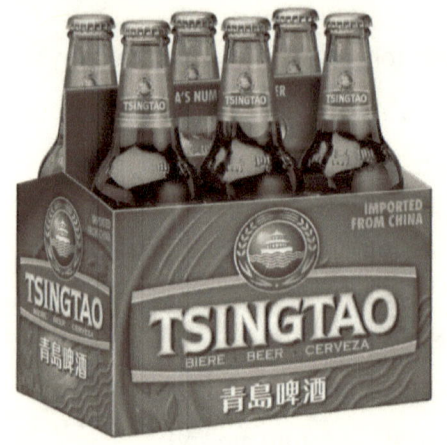

came to a stop at the museum; they could hardly wait to lay their hands on a few drinks and quench their stubborn thirsty for ethanol.

"Welcome to Tsingtao beer museum. This is the birth place of the world famous beer, Tsingtao beer. This beer is made nowhere else in the world. All the beer exported worldwide comes from this factory. Qingdao city has the purest water in the world suitable for the chemistry of this beer. Tsingtao beer has won several international awards for the best beer in the world.

The factory was founded by German settlers in 1903. The Germans occupied Qingdao in 1897-1914. The first beer was served on December 22, 1904. And hundred years on, this factory has remained in operation turning out the finest beer in the world. Tsingtao beer was introduced to the United States in 1972, and soon became the top-selling Chinese beer in the U.S market. This beer is sold in over sixty countries worldwide and accounts for more than 50% of Chinese beer exports," Snow explained

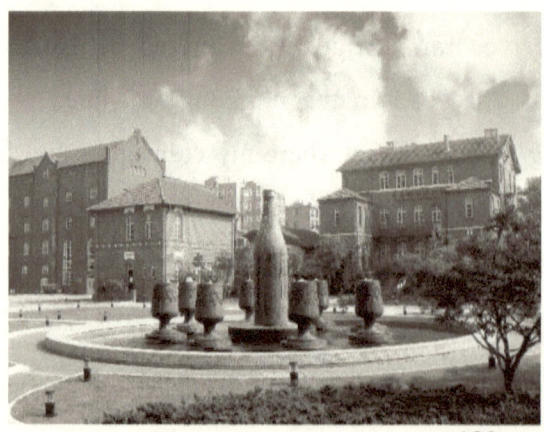

while leading her entourage through various sections of the museum.

With every word Snow used to describe the beer, the surgeons' throats burnt with yearning for a few drops to quench their thirst.

She led us through the old refinery and showed our entourage the hundred year old German pumps made by Siemens that where still operational. It was testimony of enduring German engineering. After several turns in the labyrinth of the old factory, now called the museum, the passages opened to a wide beer tasting foyer.

"This explains why most of the restaurants we saw on our way here have German names," the Emperor explained emptying his third glass of alcohol.

"Mm," Dr Gytano nodded quietly; his mouth full of contents from the green bottle.

"If this factory had been in Africa, those foolish politicians would have pulled it down and left it in ruins. There is no continuity in African politics. Look at how proud the Chinese are. They have put behind the occupation era and turned it into an economic muscle," said Oscar emptying his sixth bottle.

Snow sat with Linda and watched the guys empty the bottles at incredible speeds. Dr James and Anna drunk quietly in one corner; Fisher sat with Emma and drunk slowly; Serena captured these moments on her camera. Georgina drunk like a man in another corner with Hercules and Mike; I amused myself with the drama before my eyes in another corner. My keen eye had spotted a set up. I waited cunningly to prove it.

"This is the best beer I have ever tasted," said Abel standing to his feet to refill a sixth glass.

"It is certainly the best beer in the whole damn earth," Charlie agreed.

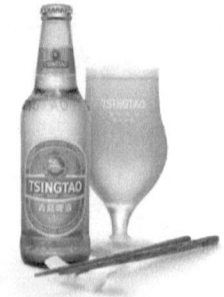

"At this stage of production, the beer is not yet pure; and not ready for export," Snow begun to explain.

I burst out laughing. Standing in my corner, I had suspected something was amiss. A group of German tourists that had gone ahead of us had disappeared in the labyrinth of the museum. I was certain; they couldn't have left this beer in a hurry without leaving glaring evidence of their exploits behind. Unless of course, sweeter beer lay yonder…

"What?" Dr Gytano asked holding a glass to his mouth.

"That's right; let's go to the next stage of the production so that you taste the real Tsingtao beer," Snow led the way smiling. The surgeons burst out laughing and staggered to their feet.

We passed a huge automated section where the beer was inspected and packed.

"In this section, over twenty five million bottles of Tsingtao beer are packed daily and ready for export," Snow explained. My fellow surgeons watched in astonishment as I was.

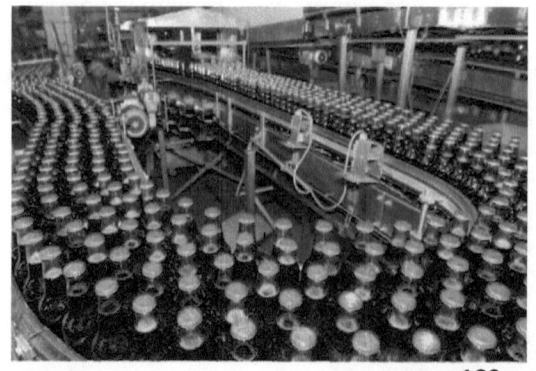

We entered the final tasting area. It was the most beautiful beer tasting club we had ever seen. A live band was there to entertain us. It was designed like an upper market night club. Several other tourists sat on tables and were drinking. I spotted the Germans holding gigantic pints in their large hands. They had come from various towns of German drawn in thousands by this green bottle, the Tsingtao beer. Their thirsty was never too early for the Qingdao international beer festival held annually in August.

The surgeons found two adjacent tables and drowned their thirsty in Tsingtao. This would be one of the most memorable moments we would hold our entire life. Fisher drunk with Serena and Emma; Linda couldn't help but taste this golden clear liquid. Georgina drunk like a Pro; Esther too couldn't be left out. I chose to join the Germans for a chit chat.

"Are you from Africa?" one asked me.

"Yes," I answered. "Southern Africa to be precise…"

"South Africa…" a big fellow holding a large glass of beer answered.

"Are you here for the Tsingtao beer too?" another asked. "Our great grandparents started this beer factory."

"You Germans love alcohol," I said. "I came to study Medicine."

"Chinese Medicine…," they burst out laughing. "Africa never ceases to amaze me; It is now turning to Chinese Medicine."

"What is wrong with you people?" a drunken looking fellow asked.

"Am studying western medicine," I tried to enlighten my visibly proud comrades.

"Western Medicine in China, you are kidding," they remarked astonished.

By 9pm, I was dead beat. It had been a long day; however the Qingdao party had just begun. My German friends showed no signs of leaving any time soon.

***

We checked into the luxurious Ocean View five star hotel at 11pm. We had a wonderful first day. Snow led us through a large gyratory door which opened into a glamorous hotel lobby. The receptionists dressed immaculately and wore pleasant smiles on their faces. I was exhausted; I couldn't wait to take a shower and fall sleep.

"You will each be provided with two cards; one is for the lift to your floor and the other is for your room. This will prevent the guys from sleep walking to the girls' rooms. The lifts can only go to your respective floors," Snow explained handing out the cards.

The surgeons laughed as they staggered towards the lifts.

***

Dawn prepared for sunrise; the Ocean turned into a silver glow and the waters sparkled like a billion diamonds when the sun rays touched them.

I awoke early the next morning. The view of the Pacific Ocean from My window on the 47th Floor of the luxurious Ocean View Hotel was mind blowing. There were several Luxurious Yachts I could see on the Ocean. I counted seventeen large ships from my room and several others docked in port. I opened the window and looked down below; the fresh ocean breeze gently caressed my face. I took a deep breath and inhaled the sweet early morning Ocean scent. I sighed as I listened to the sweet melody the giant waves made when they smashed into the coastal wall. While I listened to the whistling winds rising from the ocean, a ship sounded its loud horn as if to warn me to stay away from the window. I withdrew my head quickly and checked my safety perimeter. The view from this height was incredibly too beautiful to let fear of heights and a rogue vessel prevent me from enjoying it. I got my camera out and prepared to take incredible photos of the amazing Ocean scenery at sunrise.

The cars below looked like children's toys. The residents of this coastal city simply parked their cars along the road and any space they could find. I turned my attention to the noise on my right and saw workers loading steel onto a cargo ship. A giant barge sailed by towing a giant crane.

While I stood at the window of the elegant Ocean View five star hotel, the sun rose and cleared the darkness away. This brought the sea into clear view. I stared at the Pacific Ocean as far as the eye could see. It was so beautiful. There were several giant ships and barges on the clear blue ocean. The ships I saw at the crack of dawn, where now joined by several smaller vessels and magnificent Yachts. While I gazed, a barge sailed slowly passed my view towing a giant crane towards a large ship that was loaded with goods from distant lands. I counted over twenty smaller vessels on the ocean. Several other ships where in port. Giant anchors, resembling giant drum sticks could be seen on the shore.

While I was watching these mesmerizing scenes, all the other surgeons were glued to their windows too in their respective rooms.

***

We spent the second day in Qingdao city along the beautiful coast of the Pacific Ocean. Our Local Tour guide, Snow, took us for a hike to a mysterious Mountain. We left our tour bus at a large car park at the coast and took a local shuttle to Taiqing Mountain. We drove along a coastal road which had a beautiful view of the ocean. Snow had advised us to take seats on the right side of the bus in order to enjoy the view. However, she had not prepared us for the roller coaster ride that would come with this spectacular view. The road meandered following the twists and bends of the mountainous terrain of the coast line. The Chinese driver at the wheel drove his bus at full speed sending his passengers into suppressed mourns and screams. The experience was like a roller coaster ride.

Esther thought the driver had been hired to kill us. Several other tourists shared the bus with us.

We arrived at Taiqing Mountain safely. Linda and the girls could breathe a sigh of relief. Snow decided to take us to visit the Mysterious 2000 year old Taiqing Temple. The entrance was guarded by a giant gate.

"The giant gate in the middle is used by emperors; we will have to take the side gates," Snow explained when we got to the ancient entrance.

"No, we want to go through the main gate," Dr Hercules said and let out his splendid burst of laughter.

"Snow, Dr Abel is Emperor Selassie. Open the royal gate for him," remarked Bob Jr. pointing at Dr Abel Selassie. Everyone burst out laughing. Snow led the medical tourists through the side gates. She loved the group's sense of humor. It made her feel deeply part of the group.

"Taiqing palace is the oldest, largest and best preserved temple located on Laoshan, in Qingdao city. Laoshan Mountain is a famous scenic spot of China. It has an area of 440 square kilometers. Many Taoists once cultivated themselves here. Among various Taoist buildings on the mountain, the Taiqing Palace has the longest history. The Laoshan Taiqing Palace was first built in 140 B.C.

During the Yuan Dynasty, 1271-1368, the temple became a Taoist temple of Quanzen Sect. It got great support from the imperial court and its status was elevated greatly. Famous Toaoist Zhang Sanfeng once cultivated himself here during the Ming Dynasty, 1368-1644.

In total, there are 140 rooms and halls inside Taiqing Palace, including three Emperors' Hall, three gods hall and others. The palace was built around 2000 years ago during the reign of the first emperor of the Northern Song Dynasty and was completely renovated during the Ming Dynasty, around 500 years later.

One of the best sites, I will show you at the Palace is the clear blue pool in front of the three Purities hall," Snow explained in her beautiful accent.

"Snow, is this pool 2000 years old too?" Dr Hercules asked.

"This pool is called Shengshui spring and is believed to have never dried up for 2000 years," Snow answered smiling.

"Do you believe that too, Snow?" Dr Abel asked.

Snow smiled and continued leading the group through a maze of passages and stairs. After a few turns, we came to the famous 2000 year old Pool.

"These religious scripts were written by Kublai Khan, the first Emperor of the Yuan Dynasty, and Genghis Khan. There is also a giant stone located in the palace with four Chinese words engraved in large characters; Boi Hi can Tian, meaning; 'the waves reach to the sky'," Snow explained. "In the past, people visiting the pool used to drink this water in the belief that it would bring them good fortune. These days, people throw coins in the pool hoping a blessing would come their way. The water is no longer safe to drink anymore just in case Abel would like to take a sip from this 2000 year old pool. It is not a Fountain of youth."

"This is the water used to make Tsingtao beer. It tastes like alcohol. Taste it Dr Selassie," said Dr Hercules laughing.

The group laughed. Snow's sense of humor was venerable as was her beauty. While in Guangzhou, we had been told about a wonderful tour guide we would find in Qingdao. Snow turned out to be more than words had attempted to describe her. She was so adorable that everyone immediately fell for her; including Serena and Emma.

She showed us several trees that were over 800 years old at the Temple ground and another that was over 1000 years old. Several other Tourists with their guides were already at the Temple.

After an enlightening botanical tour, the group emerged into a large courtyard. There were large sculptors of the gods. Three gods sat on thrones and stared at the visitors with palpable expressions on their faces.. Snow explained the three gods; the god of earth, the god of heaven and the god of water.

"Hideous Idols, I don't want to look at them," Esther remarked.

"This is the era of religious tolerance. You can't say that at other people's gods and way of worship," Gytano rebuked her.

Several Chinese tourists, who were there burnt incense to the gods and begged for various blessings;

Linda wondered how her God in Heaven felt about this place she was visiting. The earth god didn't look too pleased with his Job. He had the most terrifying facial expression of the three gods. His eyes bulged from their sockets as if he suffered from Thyrotoxicosis; a debilitating endorcrine disorder.

"This is the god you come to invoke when your neighbor annoys you," said Mike loudly.

"He looks like a very stern and ruthless judge of the middle kingdom," Oscar agreed.

"I want to jump inside and grab some fruits from these gods; looks like someone is over feeding them. Just look at those big bananas, oranges and Peach," said Dr Hercules.

"I want to take a photo with the god of earth," said Charlie.

"No, you shouldn't enter their court. Remember the tour guide forbade us from taking photos with these gods," Dr Gytano reminded Hercules and Charlie.

"These are merely idols; I am not bound to respect them," Dr Hercules replied.

"We live in an Era of religious tolerance my friend. Learn to respect and accommodate other people's beliefs. If they believe in these three gods, who are you to condemn them?" Dr Gytano cautioned his friends.

While Dr Gytano Odinga preached his sermon on religious tolerance at the Taiqing Temple, Snow the tour guide led us to another ancient tree dating back to the Qing dynasty.

"There was a Famous Chinese Novelist that spent a month at this temple during the Qing dynasty. This tree here is one of the characters in his book. He depicts the tree as a beautiful girl by day that turns into a ghost by night. Here she is on the stone sculptor next to the tree," Snow explained while leading us away from the temple.

The next stop was at the fabulous old fisherman's beach. The tourists ran towards the beach excited; they took off their shoes and ran towards the blue waters of Qingdao. We played games in the dazzling white sand. The waves splashed into Hercules and Marx's legs. The two had taken to the water immediately they set foot on the beach.

***

The medical tourists spent the next day sailing on the Pacific Ocean. We set sail from the famous Olympic sailing square. It was the most delightful holiday I had to Qingdao city in Shandong province; one I would cherish for the rest of MY LIFE.

We returned from Qingdao aboard a Hainan Airlines plane. We were profoundly exhausted.

***

Marx awoke the following morning with one thing on his mind. He wanted to see Liu Lu, his Chinese girl friend. He had missed her so much and could not wait to see her. Dr Rolex, Anna and I decided to spend our afternoon on the wards of the magnificent Nafang Hospital.

Attempts to persuade Marx to come with us to the wards fell on deaf ears. He left campus to visit the medical equipment city, 100km away from his University room. He planned to meet with Liu there and discuss a business venture he was interested in. The advanced transport system in Guangzhou made travelling seem like a walk in the park. Marx selected Line 1 and directed his finger at Huadwan on the touch screen of the Automatic ticket vending machine. He collected his one pass ticket and descended down the earth by an escalator to reach the platform of line three. This trip cost him only three Yuan. There were a total of eight Lines on the Guangzhou Metro system buried deep beneath the earth's surface. In some places, these 100 meter long, high speed trains, ran at depths of greater than 200 meters beneath the earth's surface.

Marx stood on the platform of Jingxi Nafang Hospital wondering whether this technology would ever reach his country. The distance between his city and the capital was 500km and took six to eight hours to travel. His town was a tourist capital and one of the most visited cities in the whole of southern Africa. The city was home to one of the seven natural wonders of the world, the Victoria Falls. 'A high speed train would cut the distance between the two cities to only an hour. The returns this would bring to the various businesses and the travelling public would be immense,' Marx thought to himself.

While Marx's mind thought these things, his train arrived. On line three as on many other lines, the underground trains ran at intervals of five minutes in rapid pursuit of each other. When the doors closed, the beautiful voice of the announcer reminded the travelers where the train was destined.

"The destination of this train is Tiyu Xilu," the voice said and repeated the same announcement in three other languages Marx could not understand. In his mind's eye, he could see the announcer smiling as she spoke. He could even see her incredible beautiful Chinese figure.

At Yantang, two stations from Jingxi, Marx changed trains and got on to line six that would take him to his final interchange with line 1 at Dongshankou. He walked through a maze of escalators that lowered him deep below the earth's surface and at times pulled him out of the depth of the earth. A sea of Chinese people, each minding his own business, was all around him. Marx felt very safe in the company these millions of Chinese travelling with him through the belly of the earth. He had never come across so numerous a people that were as wonderful as Angels. If race could be traded, Marx would have gladly become Chinese at that very moment.

He stood on the train and supported himself by holding to a rail attached to the roof of the train. There was no limit to the number of people these trains could carry, provide one could find a space to stand and balance themselves without falling over while the trains raced at the speed of sound for the next station ahead.

As the train cruised toward Martyr's park, Marx allowed his mind to play a game he and his friends used to love in medical school. Many years had passed since, however he found the game still exhilarating. The game was called spot diagnosis. It involved looking at a person or patient and assigning a diagnosis without having to take a history or examining the subject. Marx was quick to note that, in china, Trisomy 21 could play with an iphone 6 with easy and write advanced text using mandarin characters. There were also numerous Chinese people with eyes just like those of Africans and Europeans. Marx was convinced had his school mates been present with him; they would have added Cretinism and Achondroplasia to the list of possible diagnosis on the train. In both of these conditions, the sufferers face serious vertical challenges. Marx stood at 1.88 meters and could easily reach the rails above for support; however he was dwarfed by numerous Chinese men on the train. 'These tall guys must be from the North of China,' he thought to himself. Marx then turned to his specialty; beauty diagnostics. He challenged his mind to spot all the cute ladies on the train.

Every where he looked, he was surrounded by beauty his eyes had never seen before in flesh and blood. He was not sure whether to agree with one traveler who wrote; 'they are endowed with beauty of Angels in bodies of seduction and sin.'

The train loaded its cars with more passengers at every Station they came to. It would stop for five minutes, slide open it's automatic doors to swallow this never ending swam of commuters. The crowding on the train swell as it left Chen Clan Academy metro station. Marx found himself pinned against an extraordinary beautiful lady and the side of the train. She smiled candidly when their eyes met. She didn't seem to mind the fact they were pressed against each other face to face. Her breasts firmly pressed onto Marx's lower chest. He leaned backward slightly in order not to cause her breast pain. She said something in Chinese looking at him. Unfortunately he could not catch a thing she said. However, he reasoned whatever it was she said, it required, 'you are welcome' for an answer.

***

Linda awoke early on her last Sunday in China and the beautiful city of Guangzhou. Her mind was clear on how to spend this special Sunday. She would join Dr Hercules and Dr Charlie for church that met at the prestigious Hilton hotel in the central business area of Guangzhou. She called Hercules on his cell to ask him whether she could go with him as she didn't know the way.

"Dr Hercules, please don't leave me. I would like to join you for church this morning," Linda spoke to Dr Hercules on phone.

"I am sorry Doc; I am afraid I have already left campus for church. You could come with Dr Charlie, he knows the way," Hercules replied.

Linda was disappointed as she had wanted to attend church on her last Sunday in China. She thought for a while on what to do. She thought of contacting Dr Charlie but decided not to call him. She was aware he had gone out, as was his habit, with Drs Mike, Obi and Junior to an up class, late night Irish club. There was an important celebration, the commemoration of the birth of the United Nations on 24th October; they had to attend at the Taiwanese restaurant the previous night.

After thinking for a while, she decided to go by herself. She got on to the Metro station and boarded the underground train headed for Linhexi Metro station. She was the only black person on the train that morning. As always, the subway was busy. There were over a million Chinese destined for various places in Guangzhou city. She stood holding to a rail attached to the roof for support. Her train stopped for five minutes at Guangzhou east rail station before speeding off for its destination to Panyu Square. Linda exited the train at the next station, Linhexi and after a series of elevators; she emerged to the surface. Outside, the weather was hot and humid. Linda hated the hot weather. She missed the amazing cool environment in the Metro she had left underground.

Once out of the station, she tried to figure out which way to go. She read the vague text Dr Hercules had sent her; 'at Linhexi, use exit A. when you come out of the station, walk straight for about 170m; Then when you come to a big intersection, turn left and walk for about 70m. Hilton Hotel will be on your left.'

"How very African," she murmured to herself and decided to find Hilton her own way.

While Linda was looking for the way from Linhexi Metro station, Marx left his room to meet up with his Chinese girl friend. She had wanted to go with him to his Catholic church. However he was not in any mood for church that Sunday. Instead he planned to take her out to a beautiful park he had seen in central business area. He wanted to show her a man made waterfall he had seen that reminded him about the Victoria Falls in Southern Africa. He read her Wechat text and smiled to himself;

"Good morning my handsome African Man; I am free now; let us go to the church you told me about in Yide Lu," She wrote.

Marx looked at the text and smiled. He thought of a sermon he would preach to her. Several questions ran through his mind as he searched for a sermon; "What do you tell a beautiful Chinese girl about heaven when she was surrounded by heaven here in china. What do you tell her about one God when she had three gods already. How do you preach the trinity to her when she already has three gods and three emperors?" he thought. What could he tell her about human history, when her people's history could be traced to more than 5000 years? How could he promise her a better life when she was already living that same good life?"

He came to only one conclusion; he would show her love. It was the only sermon he knew how to preach. It was love she would never forget; the Dr Marximillian love. He exited the western gate of southern medical university and walked towards the Metro station at Jingxi. When he reached Walmart supermarket, just before the station, he found a Chinese man with three monkeys. He amused the crowds that had gathered around him with some tricks his monkey comrades could do. Marx decided to stop and watch the performance.

This was an all male troop. Their faces were red, unlike the dark faced monkeys Marx had seen in his Southern African region. These had thick golden brown coats of fur and very short tails. "These are Chinese baboons," Marx thought to himself.

While Marx was still studying this troop's strange features, their handler called out in a commanding voice of a kung Fu master; the monkeys sprung up and stood like soldiers on parade. The crowd was thrilled. A little boy, in a blue T shirt and black trousers stood behind the monkey man completely ecstatic. A man, in a blue shirt and gray trousers stood next to the boy held his mouth in total amusement. A beautiful young lady, stood with her hands wrapped around the waist of her boy friend totally amused by the performance. She wore tightly fitting jeans shorts and a white top that exposed her belly button. She rested her head on her boyfriend's left shoulder and hooked her right leg against his left leg. It was a performance Marx found much more mesmerizing than the monkey tricks he was watching. This was not a new sight to Marx. He had observed keenly ever since he landed in china, the girls of Guangzhou were passionate tactile lovers. They clung to their boyfriends like climber plants do to a strong tree for support. They did not hide their feelings. They kissed publicly, walked holding each other visibly and deeply in love. "Maybe this intensity of love is resulting from a deep longing for a brother they never had," Marx thought to himself while crossing the busy pedestrian crossing, opposite Jing Hua Hotel, and walked fifteen meters towards Jingxi metro station entrance C.

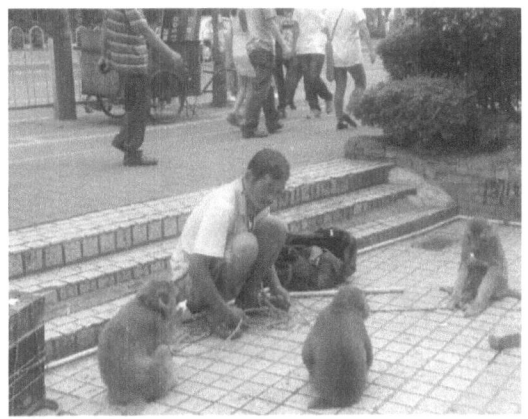

The girls of Guangzhou, including older women dressed incredibly sexy. A typical African traveler would totally misunderstand this extremely revealing attire to be a sign of sexual desire. Marx was fortunate to learn this early; women here were very proud of their bodies and enjoyed to show off their beauty just like flowers enjoy blossoming in the sun. They were like love birds proudly celebrating their beautiful feathers with song. The Chinese girls are like roses. They were China's national symbol of beauty in his mind.

Dr Marx observed that in China, women had attained dress freedom their counterparts in many African countries and Islamic states could only dream about. Women in Africa heaped layers upon layers of clothing to conceal their dark bodies despite the hot climates they lived in. Many Chinese men found the giant African woman completely undesirable in the face of their Chinese beauties all around them.

Marx hypothesized that; too much clothing formed an incubating chamber, causing the women to grow giant bodies. They were like giant sweet potatoes buried in the ground and cut from the sun light above. The resulting giant bodies were simply trying to break free and find their way to the world outside. Could it be the reason our women look bloated up? Dr Marx questioned the hypothesis that had formed in his medical mind as he boarded his train to Zhujiang.

Meanwhile at Linhexi, Linda had found her way to Hilton. She walked straight ahead when she exited the station. There were spectacular sky scrapers all around her built out of glass walls. They shined majestically in the morning sunlight. Linda passed the magnificent China plaza. Men suspended on ropes where cleaning its glass walls high above in the sky. They looked like tiny objects from where she stood. She walked on until she reached a big intersection Hercules text may have referred to. Just across, she noticed several magnificent Hotels towering towards the sky above; Star Hotel, Jianguo hotel next to an artificial water fall. There was no sign of Hilton Hotel anywhere. The poster in front of her was written in Chinese. She could only make out Chunjianghui and Star Hotel above the poster. She tried to look for any person carrying a bible. But again, this was china. 'They probably have bible apps installed on their smart phones and tablets,' she thought.

She took a Left turn just in front of Star Hotel, at the large intersection and walked along Linhe Xiheng Lu, reading every poster on the way. She passed the Cosmetic Surgery Hospital on her left and walked on.

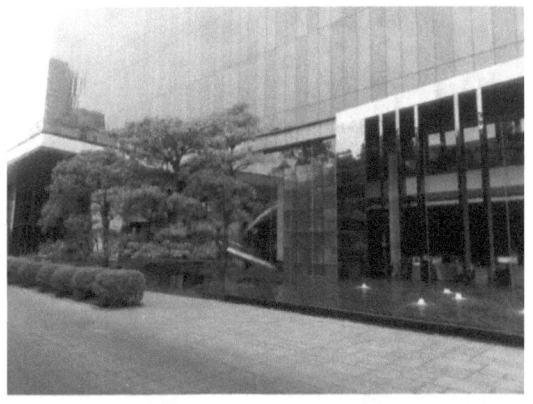

Hilton hotel was beyond her wildest imagination. It was an imposing multi storey glass sky scraper. It comprised of four sections that looked like they had been suspended on top of each other from the ground where Linda stood. She stood for a while admiring the large water fountain in front of the Hotel and a little forest garden near the entrance. Several guests sat outside on the hotel terraces sipping coffee, Chinese tea and drinking alcohol.

Linda worked her way through the magnificent hotel lobby and got on a lift that took her to the third floor. Once on the third floor, she approached an American to ask for direction to the conference room where the church conducted its service.

"Excuse me, could you please show me where believers meet for fellowship," she asked.

"You are welcome sister, Brother Peter will show you the way," he answered pointing at a big black man standing next to him.

"Come with me my sister. Where are you from?" brother Peter asked with a deep Nigerian accent.

"I am from Zambia," Linda answered.

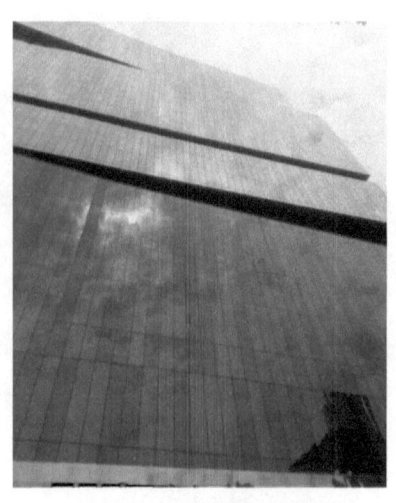

"Zambia shall be Free. I love your country, it is very peaceful," he answered with reference to a book title by Kenneth Kaunda, Zambia's first president.

Brother Peter led Linda into a wide auditorium where they found several people singing praise songs. She thanked Brother Peter and worked her way to the front to get a seat. She spotted Dr Hercules in the second row clapping and singing along.

A lady with European features stood at the pulpit and told the congregation her missionary work at an orphanage in rural China. She talked about the beautiful little children that had been abandoned by their families because of being handicapped or due to incurable diseases some children suffered.

"…..there are many children at the orphanage; many of whom are handicapped" she explained. "There is one I would like to tell you about; Little Emily. She was given to us under special circumstances. She was only twenty days old at the time. She was cute and lovely. We were delighted to have her. However, we soon found out, Emily had been diagnosed of an incurable brain tumor. We were very sad when we first received this horrible news. We were told Emily would not live to two months of age. We conducted all brain scans possible at top hospitals and all the results came back the same; Emily would die. We then turned to God and prayed. Emily is now six years old and in school. She is extremely bright and learning fast ahead of her age. God healed Little Emily. We took her back to her doctors; everyone was shocked to see Emily alive. All the recheck tests came out negative. The Brain tumor is gone. God healed Little Emily. Church God is alive and at work here in China. I urge all of you to continue praying for God's favor on China," she testified.

The church was ecstatic when they heard her story. Linda looked around and saw Dr Charlie walking in and soon took a seat next to Dr Oscar, Georgina and Dr Gytano. This was their last Sunday in China. They had come to seek blessings for the long journey ahead.

Dr Charlie would say; he was there to download a new anti sin software for his brain and to rid himself of any corruptible files in his brain with a tendency of leading him into sin, a feature he referred to as entropy.

While Linda was enjoying this fellowship, Marx arrived at Linhexi metro station and headed for the park just opposite to the station. Liu Lu, his Chinese girl friend was still on the way to meet him. He decided to pass time by inspecting an artificial water fall between Star Hotel and Jianguo Hotel. The view was spectacular. Many lovers were there ahead of Marx, they were drawn by the enchanting power this little water fall possessed.

Marx immediately 'we chatted' Liu Lu asking her to meet him at the little water fall; he wanted them to take photos like the couples he was watching had. Liu had no problem finding Marx. She was delighted to see him.

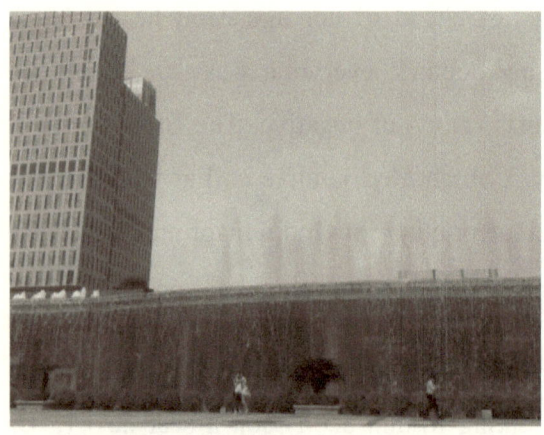

"I wanted to go with you to church in Yide Lu," she protested.

"I was not too well. I was coughing. I am still coughing actually. I got flu but nothing to worry. I wanted us to take photos in front of this waterfall," Marx explained.

"I know it reminds you of the Victoria Falls in southern Africa," she giggled.

"You know the Victoria falls. When you come to Africa, I will take you there. It is a breath taking sight. In fact it is designated as one of the natural wonders of the world," Marx explained.

"I forget the name of the European man who named it after the Queen of England, remind me his name," said Liu.

"It was Dr David Livingstone. When he visited the site in 1855, he wrote in his diary these words; 'scenes so beautiful, they must have been viewed by angels in their flight'..." Marx explained.

"Yes, I remember him now; let us go to the park, I want to sit down," she said.

They walked across to the park and found a place to sit.

"I brought Chinese medicine for your cough, you must drink it," she told him when they had sat down.

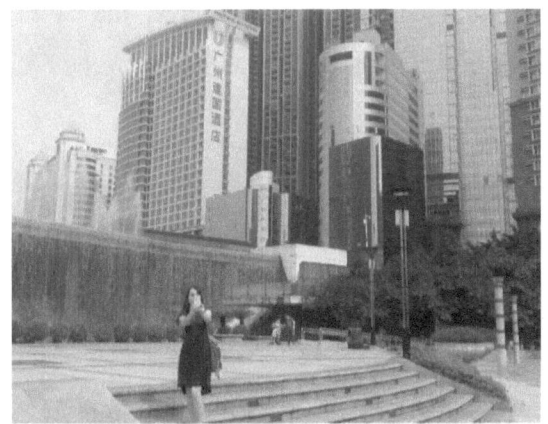

"No, I don't need any medicine, I am fine now," Marx tried to protest.

Liu pulled out a black liquid in a container from her hand bag. Curiously, Marx asked to look at the medicine bottle closely. The bottle had no label on it. He opened its lid and sniffed. It smelled awful;

"The bottle feels warm. Where did you find this terrible thing? This is 500ml, is it a sexual potency enhancing drug?" Marx asked.

"I bought it from a traditional Chinese doctor on my way to meeting you. It is warm because it has to be taken warm. Now drink it. Your cough will go, trust me. You must finish the whole bottle for the medicine to be effective," Liu explained.

"Suppose it causes me bizarre sexual appetite, what will you do?" he asked

"That's why am here, to take care of you. I won't run away like your African wife did. I will look after you," she reassured him. "However, don't think too much."

Marx wanted to refuse but changed his mind. He didn't want to disappoint his girlfriend. She was caring and thoughtful of him. 'How could I say no to such a gorgeous and considerate young lady?' He thought to himself. He opened the bottle, closed his eyes and in one swallow, he emptied the contents of the bottle down his throat.

"Oh, my God, it is awful, it is bitter. It is horrible, I am going to be sick," he moaned.

Liu laughed at him uncontrollably. She was so excited he had taken the medicine. She reached out into her hand bag and handed him some sweetened orange pills to chew.

"Here chew this, it will take away the bitterness," she said.

He grabbed the pieces of orange peels and chewed. However this did not help him.

"Give me more of this sweet stuff, oh this medicine is terrible. Do people really drink this stuff? It is horrible," he complained.

"I gave you poison. You will die. It will make you sleep then I will sell you," she said laughing.

Marx wished he had followed his colleagues to the Church at Hilton. He wouldn't have suffered the decree of this terrible prescription.

***

Meanwhile at church, the pastor came up the pulpit and begun to teach;

"Who are we supposed to be? The Way we follow is Not a Lifestyle; It is not Magic tricks; It is not a set of 'DOs and DON'Ts'; The aim of Magic tricks is to fool people, to deceive people; The way we follow is not a form of religion, it is Power by the name of Jesus Christ; We live in a world of many philosophies. The Holy Spirit produces fruits in us. Which are; love, joy, peace, patience, kindness, goodness, faithfulness, gentleness, and self-control? Against such things there is no Law. You can read about this in Galatians 5:22-23.

Paul; when he stood for trial before Felix said these words in Acts 24:14; 'However, I admit that I worship the God of our fathers as a follower of the WAY, which they call a sect.'

The Way is Lifestyle of love; the Way is revelation and teaching by the Holy Spirit, The Way is Power.

Jesus said; I am the Way. John 14:6" The pastor concluded his brief sermon and called the meeting to a close. The choir rose and sung a closing song. A beautiful Chinese girl played the guitar. She wore a red top and a tight black trousers; a white male song leader, who looked like Keith Green, led the singers. He wore a black T shirt, jeans trousers and orange shoes. There were two black singers in this band.

Linda thought of how she had looked for the Way to Hilton that morning as she left the magnificent hotel hosting the congregation she had visited. On the way, she wondered whether the Holy Spirit had been teaching her something about finding Jesus in China. She thought about the many Chinese temples she had visited, including the 2000 years old Taiqing temple in Qingdao. She was convinced Chinese people where a deeply religious society. She admired them for their religious devotion. They had invented three gods in their quest to find the Way. And for thousands of years, they closed themselves from the outside world.

While she thought these things, she ran into bro. Peter.

"Anyone wishing to know about world power should study the history of Israel and the founding of the United States of America," he said.

"If only they would know the Way, they would find Real Power that Conquers the World. The Way would satisfy their tempestuous hearts," Linda answered. "God has always used powerful nations to spread his word or to bring judgment on a sinful nation. The Roman Empire, British Empire and the United States ruled the world because they put their Trust in God. America has abandoned God and is quickly losing its grip on world dominance. It has become a nation of heathens," said Brother Peter with a deep Nigerian Accent.

"This is probably China's time to rule the world," said Linda

"But that can only happen if they embrace the one true God of heaven. America has lost the Way; the Chinese have the opportunity to find the way now. The power over the world is given to those who find the way," said Dr Hercules who had joined Linda and Brother Peter.

"It is not in Armies or Number of nuclear arsenals. If the Chinese miss the way and put their trust in the Economy and Army they will never rule the world; Armies and Economic boom can easily crumble," said Brother Peter.

"It takes only confusion in the army and volatility in the economy and their dream for world dominance will slip off their fingers for another one thousand years," said Hercules.

"They will recoil to being a closed, warring middle kingdom of ancient times. All the development they have scored in the last sixty years will crumble around them," said Linda.

"We must pray for China to rule the world. It is a true friend of Africa. The Chinese people do not know racial discrimination. Africans are welcome here. They treat Africans as equals," Brother Peter answered.

"Personally, there are times when I have even forgotten I was African. The Chinese made me feel at Home. I think Africa should have discovered China earlier," said Linda

"Even now, it is not too late. You and I are privileged to be here and discover this genuine friendship China is extending to Africa. China is Africa's hope for development. She is indeed Africa's 'all weather' friend," Dr Hercules observed.

"Sister, Zambia shall be Free. China and Africa shall Rule the world," said Brother Peter as they came to the pedestrian crossing towards Linhexi Metro station.

Am Ready to Go

I walked down the beautiful terraces of the David Livingstone Safari Lodge, down to the river bank. The view of the Zambezi River was breath taking. The amazing spray at the Victoria Falls was clearly visible in the distance. I spotted a school of hippos on long island just across from where I stood.

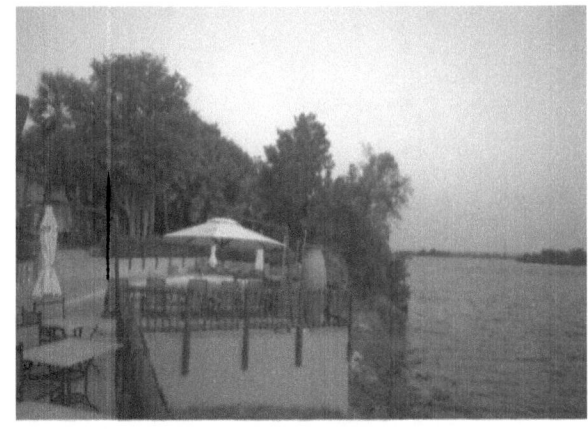

I was at David Livingstone Safari Lodge to set up an Emergency clinic for delegates attending a G-8 committee of Heads of State Summit. My responsibilities were colossal. Several African heads of state would be attending this five day summit. Our country's President was scheduled to open the meeting later that day. Security presence was heavy and the mood tense. However, I found time to relax at the magnificent swimming pool built on the river bank. The blue water inside the pool beckoned me to dive in and swim while running through a list of medical conditions that could rain down on the clinic at a summit like this. I sighed and let my mind search for the worst case scenario. I reflected on the circumstances that led to the death of one of our gallant president in a resort town, Sharm El Sheikh, in Egypt while attending a Heads of states summit.

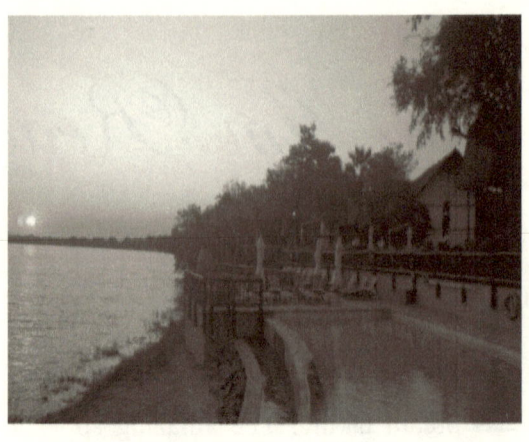

Sharm el-Sheik is an Egyptian resort town between the desert of Sinai Peninsula and the Red Sea. It is known for its sheltered sandy beaches, clear waters and coral reefs. Naama Bay, with a palm tree-lined promenade, is filled with bars and restaurants.

I didn't like this part of my work.

While I thought these things, a Lady I recognized meeting at the hospital walked over to where I stood. She was immaculately dressed and carried herself with a disposition of someone entrusted with heavy responsibility.

"Hello doctor," she greeted me. "I am pleased to see you here. Are you here for this summit?"

"I am here for the clinic. The rooms we have been given are too far away from the conference room. It is too far in an event of a Heart attack or a Stroke. We should have set close by. Unfortunately we were not consulted on the set up. I just learnt of the clinic today," I complained.

"That's too bad. Did you know I worked here? Do you remember me?" the lady asked.

"Yes Mrs. NK. I remember you from the hospital; Fridah's sister," I answered.

"I thought you wouldn't recognize me. Too bad about the rooms; the people that came to book for the rooms didn't tell us what you are saying; I don't think they even understood the importance of location. I am in-charge of reservation at the Lodge."

"I didn't know there was such a beautiful paradise here in Livingstone. Please book me for a weekend here. I love this place. It is my first time to be here."

"You are most welcome doc. You will definitely enjoy yourself, especially the late afternoon boat cruise to experience the enchanting sunset on the Zambezi. We are a Five Star Lodge and internationally recognized. Now doc, a quick one; it's about my husband. You were with him when he left. I have tried to imagine how it was. Please tell me about it."

I thought for a while and recalled the events. I remembered how in his frailty, he had stared impassively in the distance. Something only he could see drew all his attention to gaze on. There was no struggle or foaming at the mouth. There were no secretions of gall from his nostrils. No heavy laboured breathing or a rage of fits; he simply gazed in the distance. He looked like someone that had been called; it was as if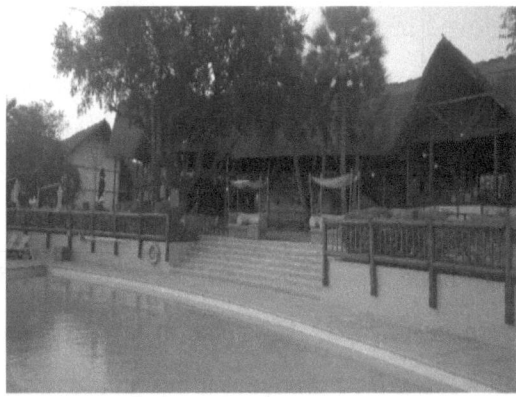

he were in a trance, watching the host of heaven riding by in his fiery chariots. He had come to pick him. I could almost hear him mumble something to his wife in the words of a poet;

Mr. NK had been taken ill without warning on 30th October, 2014. He had been well all day the previous day and was even tending to his garden at home. He had developed sudden severe abdominal pain and was rushed to Surgical Tourism City Hospital where I worked. We gave him a diagnosis of intestinal obstruction. Now, this condition is said to occur when the intestines fail to propel their contents distally due to a mechanical obstruction. When this happens, patients experience severe abdominal pain and many would start vomiting bile. They would not pass wind or stool. Their blood pressure may plummet while the pulses soar high. They may become sweaty and anxious.

On arrival at the hospital he was immediately admitted to surgical ward and prepared for surgery. Our surgical team planned to conduct an exploratory laparatomy following failure at attempts for decompression. A Nasal Gastric tube had been inserted via his right nostril down his stomach. Dark bilious secretions drained down into the containing bag on the side of the bed. His wife, heavy with child, anxiously looked on as her beloved friend groaned in pain. She wished the doctors could quickly find the cause of the obstruction in his intestine and allow them to go home.

However, this obstruction would not resolve spontaneously. Mr. NK was finally wheeled to the operating theatre the following day. There was high hope among his family that he would be fine once the operation had been performed. His sister in-law, worked at the hospital. There was no glint of worry that anything could go wrong. Fridah herself, was an accomplished midwife. She got along well with everyone at the hospital and she had confidence in her hospital's surgical department. She reassured her family and brother in-law, everything would turn out just fine.

The department of surgery was glad to have a visiting surgeon, Dr Mansa Ngiso, from University Hospital. He was highly competent at bowel surgery. The team was sure, in his hands, this surgery would be a walk in the park.

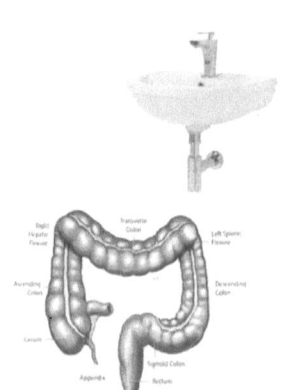

However, the finding in the abdomen was a shock to everyone, including myself. I was keenly watching the operation in theatre that day.

No sooner did the surgeon open the abdomen than he was greeted by a grossly distended ceacum. The ceacum is where the Small intestine joins the large intestine. It is a blind pouch and continues upwards as the ascending colon. The appendix is a small blind ended pouch which extends from the ceacum. The ceacum is designed much like the syphon on most kitchen sinks.

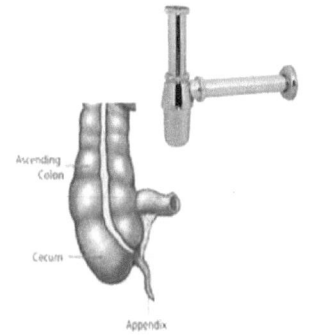

The horizontal arm or pipe would represent the small intestine joining the ceacum; the bulged lower end of the vertical limb or pipe in the picture. The point where the two join, the vertical and the horizontal pipes, would be the ileal- ceacal junction and is controlled by a one way valve; the ileal-ceacal valve. The rest of the vertical loop represents the ascending colon. The appendix would be found extending as a small blind pouch from the bottom of the ceacum. This confluence is an amazing feat of engineering made in heaven.

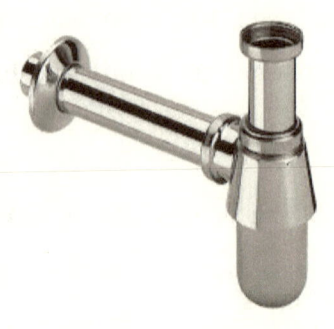

Where as in the kitchen water flows passively down the vertical limb to drain away; in the human body however, contents of bowel flows actively up stream. Intestines are lined by powerful muscles that propel this content up the ascending colon.

The findings at operation revealed that these conscientious muscles had failed to push the contents of the ceacum and ascending colon forwards resulting in a perilous bulge of the ceacum. When the syphon of the kitchen sink is blocked, water floods inside the sink and unless something is done fast, it soon flows down the floor. Similarly, the findings on the operation table were that of the effects of a flood. There was a back flow of bowel contents. However, the one way valve at the ileal-ceacal junction closed tightly resulting into a rise of pressure within the ceacum to dangerous levels. The operating surgeons found the ceacum torn at its widest point and spilled its toxic contents into the abdominal cavity.

"Doc, there is a hard mass blocking the ascending colon just below the liver," Dr Mansa explained looking up from the table.

"Does it feel like it can be resected? Does it feel to be within the lumen of the colon? Is it a polyp?" I asked a barrage of questions.

"Let me explore its full extend....," replied Dr Mansa.

While Dr Mansa explored, the cause of the obstruction, I ran through a list of the usual suspects that could cause an obstruction such as the one the Team was grappling with.

A twist in the ceacum itself could do this as well as a twist in the transverse colon; phenomena called volvulus. I prayed this should turn out a volvulus. Our team was highly competent to deal with a volvulus anywhere on large or small bowel. One hour went by but the team could not figure out the origin of the mass. It was heavily obscured from view and had numerous large blood vessels surrounding it. It was wired like a bomb. The team worked desperately like a bomb squad trying every trick in the book to diffuse a nuclear bomb.

By now, the stand by nurse, referred to as runner, had wiped Dr Mansa's sweaty face fifteen times. It was getting hot on the table. He asked for the air condition to be turned on. The Heat of Livingstone City and the Tumor had conspired against Dr Mansa. They were determined to frustrate him and were poised to succeed in hindering his desperate search for the root of this savage mass.

I ventured further search in my Medulla Oblongata's Google Scholar, PubMed, Medline and the Cochrane library for the other possible causes; I didn't like what my search uncovered; 'Colon cancer is the second commonest cause of cancer related deaths after lung cancer worldwide.'

And when finally Dr Mansa admitted defeat, shivers ran down my spine like a bout of lightning.

"Doc, this mass is extending across the abdomen to the left side up to the splenic flexure. It is fixed to the posterior abdominal wall. It is not mobile and is highly vascular. I can't even appreciate the liver. It is obscured from view. The omentum and the transverse colon are firmly adhered to it. I think this is a Cancer. It is impossible to figure out where it is arising from. I can't reach his pancreas. Looks like even the inferior vena cover is infiltrated; if we push our search further, we might tear the vena cava and we would lose the patient on the table. A left Hemi colectomy will not be possible. I am afraid we have to settle with a ceacostomy. It is not the best of stoma to make, but as things stand, it is our best option and his best chance for survival out of this theatre," Dr Mansa concluded his search and called off the exploration for a way around the savage mass.

The team was very sad. This was not what we had hoped for. The symptoms where of sudden onset and did not add up with the findings in the abdomen. Cancers usually present with gradual symptoms. However in medicine, this sudden onset of cancer complication was possible. The cancer must have been hiding out in the abdomen and stalked Mr. NK for several months before suddenly unleashing its cruelty, to cause intestinal obstruction. I wondered what could have been the Missing Link to an early discovery of this wicked tumor.

We left theatre like warriors vanquished in war. This was our friend's brother in law and the diagnosis we had arrived at would be like delivering a jury's death verdict. I walked comforting myself with hopes for a second look at which time I hoped to externalize a loop of small bowel to divert the fecal stream. The ceacum as a point of fecal stream diversion was associated with many complications. However, I was convinced there would be no next time. It was a miracle, he was still alive.

When the elevator reached the ground floor, I met Fridah. She was on the way out of the lift from second floor, the gynecology floor. She was alone and made it easy for me to explain the theatre findings. Fridah was a rational and practical person. She could take anything thrown at her. We quickly found a place to sit down and discuss how to break the news to her sister. She was eighty months pregnant. I was concerned this bad news would send NK's wife into premature labour.

"That is too bad. I wonder how my poor sister will take this news," said Fridah when we had sat down.

"Cancer was the least of our differential diagnosis," I said.

"Maybe if you had been the one operating you would have removed it," said Fridah.

"No dear, I couldn't have. I was there on the operating table, I saw the horrible tumor," I replied.

"It is inoperable. How long do you reckon he has left to be alive? I feel very sad for my sister. Do you know she is eight months pregnant? I wish he hadn't impregnated her," Fridah bemoaned.

NK's wife was anxiously waiting to hear the good news about the operation. She was certain the operation had gone well. However the news from theatre was like a scene in a bad dream. Such things happen during nightmares. They couldn't be happening in her life.

".....will he be alright?" NK's wife asked Dr Mansa.

Fridah and I had just walked into ward one. I was happy my colleague had already broken the grisly news to Mrs. NK. Fridah took over from where the team had left and led her sister to meet the nurses bringing her husband on a trolley from theatre. Several other nurses went to male surgical ward to offer their support to the two sisters.

I left the ward and strode across the car park towards the kiosk where I was met by NK's tribal cousins who ventured their own explanation into their friend's sudden illness.

"Doc, could it be the quarrel he had with his neighbor yesterday caused the obstruction you found?" one of NK's friends asked.

"No. Scientifically, that is not possible," I answered.

"You see doc, our friend had a very bad quarrel yesterday with his neighbor over a shovel he had borrowed. And when you add one and one together, this disease points to this quarrel. Remember there is no smoke without fire," Yet another of NK's friends added.

"That was merely a coincidence; what we found in Mr. NK's abdomen would have happen even without this quarrel you are referring to. Any way, we are still investigating the disease your friend has and once the pathology report is out, we will know the exact disease that has caused his sudden illness," I replied and continued on my way to the hospital kiosk.

The beautiful girls at the Kiosk; Isabel, Rebecca and Josephine greeted me but was too engrossed in my thoughts to notice.

"Doc, your bill has reached 200," Rebecca tried to get my attention.

"Don't give anyone drinks unless they have a Coca Cola prescription signed by myself," I smiled waking up from my slumber.

I got a snack at the kiosk and pondered briefly on the conversation I had with NK's friends in the car park. I was deeply disappointed by their interpretation of the cause of sudden illness in their friend. I realized there was still a long way to breaking myths and misconceptions in many people's lives. Witchcraft still had a strong grip on many people's beliefs about sickness in the community. Many still believed cancer was a disease caused by magic and witchcraft.

This belief was one of the reasons why people presented late at the hospital when afflicted by a growth on the body particularly when such growths were located on the lower limbs. Symptoms occurring in the lower limbs or legs such as; weakness, numbness, burning sensations, swelling, growths, and gangrene of the feet; were all attributed to one stepping on some charms and blamed on acts of witchcraft. As a result precious time for early presentation at the hospital would be lost and instead spent at the witchdoctor's kraal. Other diseases ending up at the witch doctor's clinic include cases of gradual abdominal and scrotal swelling.

Mr. NK was discharged from hospital in a fortnight with a colostomy. The couple was thoroughly taught how to use colostomy bags during their stay in hospital. They were glad to be finally in their house. However, this operation had greatly altered their lifestyle in the home.

Several weeks passed before I would hear from Mrs. NK. She called in the evening on Christmas Eve and asked me to explain what would be causing continued vomiting in her husband.

"Doc, my husband is vomiting a lot and appears weak. What medicine can I buy to stop him from vomiting?" She asked.

"Let me see him at the hospital immediately. Are you able to bring him right away?" I answered.

"Is it ok if we came tomorrow? You are forgetting that I am a patient too. You have all forgotten about me," she replied.

"I am terribly sorry dear. I forgot you recently had a Caesar? Tomorrow will be fine. Let me see you in casualty in the morning," I answered. I was delighted at the prospect of spending Christmas attending my patient.

"Thanks doc, we will be there in the morning. My wound is healing well, although I still experience severe abdominal pain," she replied.

A month earlier, the stress of nursing her husband gradually grew sending Mrs. NK into a complicated labour on 27th November and had to be delivered by caesarean section. She disappeared from her husband's bed side without anyone ever noticing. When her caesarean section wound was hardly 48 hours, she was back at the bed side of her beloved friend and husband. No one noticed she had gone away. During this period, I had been away from the hospital on national duties. They simply forgot she was a patient too. Even her husband did not notice. One day as she was turning him in bed, she injured her wound. He noticed and demanded to see why she was holding her abdomen in obvious distress. He could not believe what he saw and he immediately sent for her sister Fridah.

"You have been sitting by my bed side all this time when you too are a patient. Get me Fridah immediately before you kill yourself," he demanded.

She had accidentally pulled on her wound, tearing off stitches from the edge of the wound. She was in such excruciating pain that she could not hide the wound any longer from her husband. She had hid the mode of delivery from him because she didn't want him to be worrying about her considering the state he was in.

The following day on Christmas, Mr. NK was re-admitted to hospital. He was dehydrated and in obvious state of electrolyte imbalance. He was too frail to support his own weight. A wheel chair was quickly fetched to aid his locomotion. Despite his illness and frailty he was delighted to see our team. The illness had taken away his physical strength. However it had failed to take away his sense of humor.

"Doc, I want you to put back my Ass; this temporal ass you put on me is killing me. Bring back my ass," he demanded when we met in outpatient.

"How are you feeling? We will put back your ass as soon as the condition allows us," I answered with a cautious smile.

Several doctors were happy to see Mr. NK that Christmas morning. Dr Nicola admitted him to the ward after a full work up. It was December and he was anxious to have his colostomy reversed before the New Year. The couple would spend that Christmas in hospital. His wife faithfully remained at his bed side day and night. Each night, they prayed for God's Healing. He would always lay down clear plans to his wife before praying.

"Honey, here is the game plan...," he would say to his wife. "Make me a quick meal then close the curtains when I have eaten we pray."

This was their daily routine on the ward.

Mr. NK had developed a second obstruction higher up in his small bowel. His condition had deteriorated so much by now that he appeared he wouldn't make it into the New Year. Our surgical team planned an emergency surgery. I came by his bed side to assess his fitness for surgery on 29th December. He was too frail to withstand prolonged surgery. My worst fear had finally come; a second look. I doubted it would make any difference to the earlier surgery.

"Doc, where have you been? I missed you. You left me alone. I have been reading your book. I enjoy reading your writing. I hope I will be in one of your books. Have you been avoiding me?" He complained when he saw me that morning on the ward.

"No my friend; I am not avoiding you. I have been away from the hospital. I am back now," I replied feeling guilty.

"I feel good just seeing you. I am always comforted when you drop by to see me. Please pray with me," He explained looking at me.

We prayed holding hands. Then I explained I would operate on him that morning. His wife sat at his bed side. The nurses had inserted a Nasogastric tube, Intravenous lines and placed a label on his forehead. He joked and laughed in his usual humorous manner.

"I am ready to go," he said picking himself up in bed.

The porter came by shortly and soon took him into theatre. It was a Monday and the Major ward round was busy that morning, the 29th of December 2014. There were many patients on the ward being the festival season.

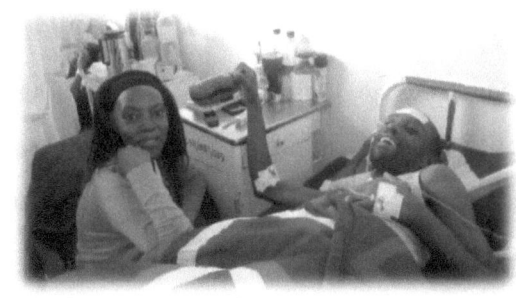

I pondered over the words Mr. NK had uttered; 'I Am Ready To Go...'

I wondered what he meant. "Is he planning to die on me in theatre?"

Hardly ten minutes into the operation than I called it off. I stared at the opened abdominal cavity in disbelief. NK's words echoed through my mind; 'I Am Ready to Go...'

"Is this what he was referring to when we spoke earlier on the ward?" I thought.

There were no intestines to be found in the abdomen. What I was looking at resembled solidified molten material. It was as if NK's inside had been melted down and the liquid poured back to solidify. It was clear in my mind; this picture was not compatible with life. I collected samples for histopathology and begun to close the abdomen. I cut out a circular window in the skin on the left side of the abdomen in the upper quadrant and pushed my finger through it. The patient had begged me to restore function at his anus; unfortunately, the cruel tumor forced me into constructing a third ass on my patient's abdomen. The tumor that Dr Mansa had fought with during NK's first operation had now invaded the entire abdomen and turned the intestines into a gigantic ball of solid molten tissue.

"It is a miracle he lived to see the birth of his lovely daughter Mapalo," I told Mr. Kalus as we left theatre.

I was met outside theatre by Mr. NK's anxious family. The news I had for them broke their hearts. His life was now in God's hands. There was nothing in the Arsenals of medical science that could be implored to reverse the findings at surgery.

Meanwhile his old pals in town, when the news about the second operation reached them, they hurried to the hospital to see their friend. However their visit was not without drama. Many were his tribal cousins and allowed themselves to indulge in talk that would otherwise be deemed taboo and inappropriate elsewhere. They began to plan a befitting send off party for him while scheming to escape the watchful eyes of their wives.

"This guy, he is not dead up to this time?" asked one of his tribal cousins.

"Why is he holding on to life this long? He must die so that we can drink lots of beers at his funeral," remarked another.

"He must die on New Year's eve so that we can officially sleep out of our homes and camp at the funeral house. Otherwise our wives won't allow us to sleep out if he continues defying and cheating death like this," yet another commented.

To everyone's amazement, Mr. NK pulled through his surgery and lived to see the New Year. A month went by and his wife continued faithfully at his bed side. She remained in high spirits and showed no signs of slowing down on her care for her husband. He was blessed to have found such a faithful wife. This truly was a woman of God talked about in proverbs; a hard working woman that loved her husband dearly; I wondered whether Fridah possessed any of these traits her sister had displayed. Her love was tasted by the blistering furnaces of life and emerged pure. Hers was truly in sickness and in health to the later. And so when one evening he asked her to spend the night at home and to leave him on the ward alone, she would not hear of it. He pleaded with her to go home to be with the children and to catch some rest. This was the only time she was ever separated from him besides the day of her caesarean section.

The next day, the fourth of week in the New Year, on the 28th day of January, Dr Nicola was on rounds and when she came to Mr. NK's bed, she noticed he was not talking. She quickly rushed to call me to check on him.

I found him staring intriguingly in the distance on the western side of the ward; He stared impassively in the distance in his frailty. Something only he could see drew all his attention to gaze on. There was no struggle or foaming at the mouth. There were no secretions of gall from his nostrils. No heavy laboured breathing or a rage of fits; he simply gazed in the distance. He looked like someone that had been called; it was as if he were in a trance, watching the Host of heaven riding by in his fiery chariots. He had come to pick him. He seemed to be saying; 'I asked my wife to spend the night at home with the kids and she is on her way right now. Could you please just wait a few minutes, she will be here. I know my wife.' I could almost hear him mumble something to his wife in the words of a poet;

Though I'm Gone, I Feel Your Love

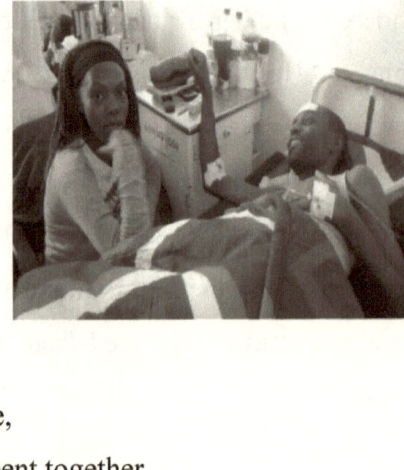

To my dear
family,
I'm sending this from
above,
That even though I'm
gone from earth,
I can still feel your love,
And all the times we spent together,
Growing a love that would last forever,
Are times that will never leave,
Because you remember me.
I'm sorry about the timing,
For I didn't want to leave,
But God called me home,
So I fell into eternal sleep.
There was so much left to do here,

Cause God took me quite young,

I had a loving family,

And so much to teach my girls.

Mapalo, you turned two months old just yesterday,

Taizya, I leave you very young at five

At sixteen, you will hardly remember my voice,

I worry what will become of you

I'm sure you all can make it,

You have God by your side,

And just to let you know,

I'm enjoying this long heavenly Harley ride.

If any of you ever need me,

Just close your eyes and I'll be there,

I'll help you through your life,

If you remember how much I cared.

I want you all to know today,

That I love you very much,

And even though I'm gone from earth,

I can still feel your love.

"This surely was a child of God; Go well my friend. Hamba Kaye."

Other books by Dr **Kelvin C Moonga**

1. **Finding Linda**
2. **The Missing Link**

    (a Cancer Awareness book based on true life accounts)
3. **I Know What You Did in China**
4. **A Few Good Doctors**
5. **Girl Child Menstrual Care & GBV Awareness Book**
6. **Women's Health in Everyday Life**
7. **When Duty Calls**
8. In the Shadow of the Great Pyramid of Giza
9. Undying Memory
10. Fatal Error
11. Curse in Court
12. Long Road to Motherhood
13. Teenage AWOL
14. CLONES
15. Game of Figs
16. Grain Shack
17. **In the Shadows of The Mighty Victoria Falls**

You can get books 1 - 7 Online. Visit amazon.com or contact Dr Kelvin C Moonga on drkmoonga2011@live.com; drkmoonga2011@gmail.com

Wechat and WatsApp # +260965868668

www.amazon.com

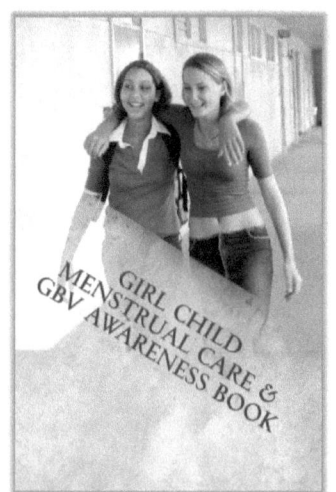

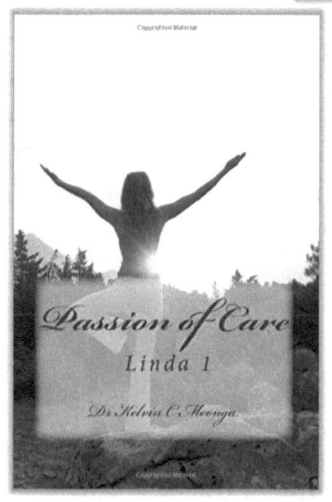

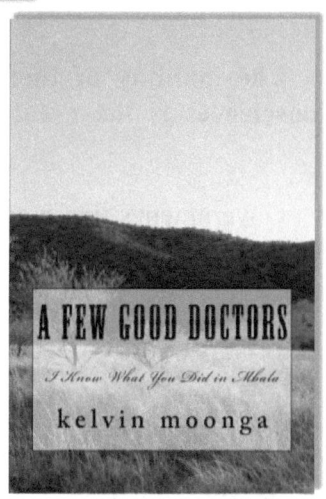

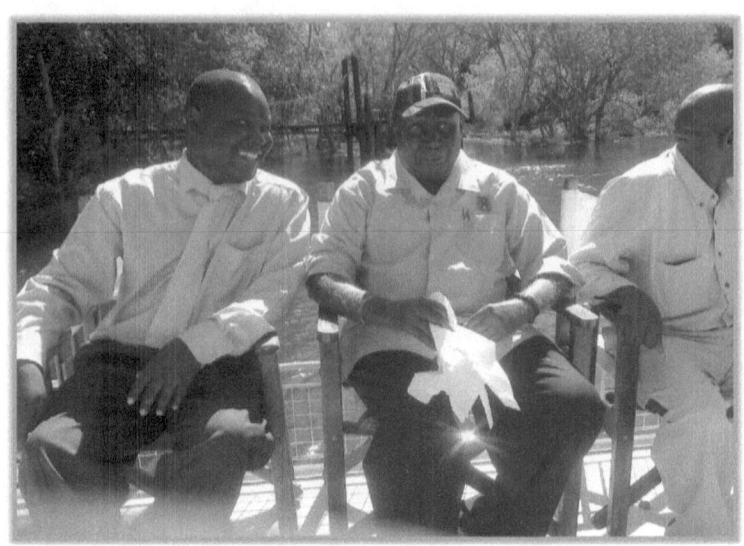

The inability of those in power to still the voices of their own consciences is the great force leading to change. **Kenneth Kaunda**

Government's first duty is to protect the people, not run their lives. **Ronald Reagan**

If your actions inspire others to dream more, learn more, do more and become more, you are a leader. -- John Quincy Adams

We, the People, recognize that we have responsibilities as well as rights; that our destinies are bound together; that a freedom which only asks what's in it for me, a freedom without a commitment to others, a freedom without love or charity or duty or patriotism, is unworthy of our founding ideals, and those who died in their defense. **Barack Obama**

With faith, discipline and selfless devotion to duty, there is nothing worthwhile that you cannot achieve. **Muhammad Ali**

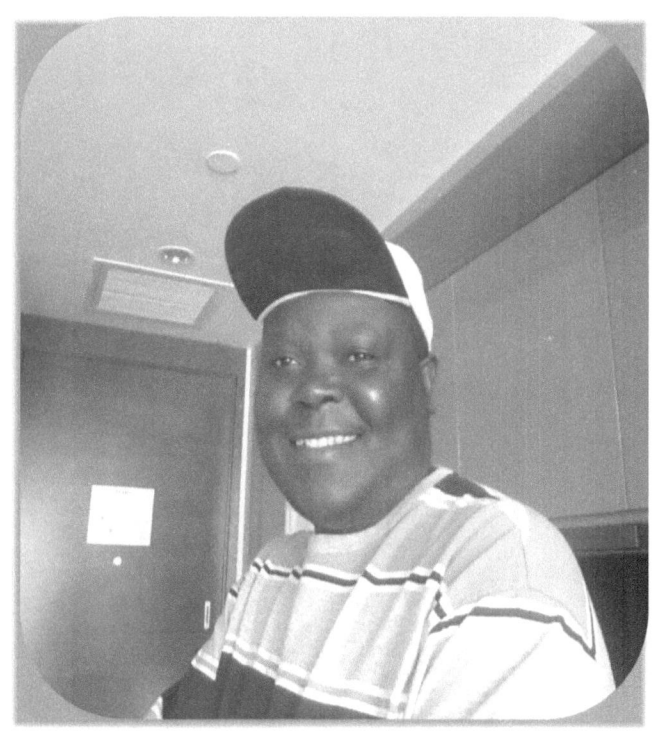

When Duty Calls, What is at Stake is Often Priceless

Dr Kelvin C Moonga